Praise for *The Pain Cure Rx*

"If you are suffering with chronic pain, this book is for you."

— **Deepak Chopra, M.D.,**
New York Times best-selling author of *The Future of God*

*"Every once in a while a book comes along that will
completely transform a field—this is that book for pain."*

— **Haylie Pomroy,**
New York Times best-selling author of *The Fast Metabolism Diet*

*"After working with Dr. Yass for so many years as an expert
for many articles in our newsletters, I am so happy to see that
he is now providing a complete guide to understanding his method
of diagnosing and treating chronic pain. I have personally shared Dr. Yass's
approach with countless people, cautioning them away from surgery and
towards the right type of exercise. None of them ended up requiring surgery!
If you are in pain, this book should be your first stop towards healing."*

— **Marjory Abrams,** Publisher of Bottom Line Publications,
the most widely read consumer newsletters ever published

THE

PAIN CURE

RX

ALSO BY DR. MITCHELL YASS

*Overpower Pain: The Strength-Training Program
That Stops Pain Without Drugs or Surgery*

THE

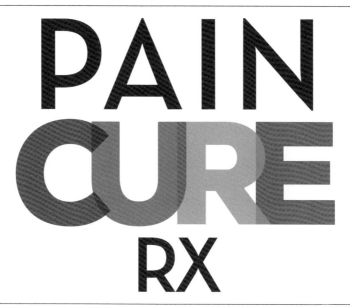

PAIN CURE RX

THE YASS METHOD
FOR DIAGNOSING AND
RESOLVING CHRONIC PAIN

DR. MITCHELL YASS

HAY HOUSE, INC.
Carlsbad, California • New York City
London • Sydney • Johannesburg
Vancouver • Hong Kong • New Delhi

Copyright © 2015 by Inky Dinky Worldwide, Inc., and Mitchell Yass

Published and distributed in the United States by: Hay House, Inc.: www.hayhouse.com® • *Published and distributed in Australia by:* Hay House Australia Pty. Ltd.: www.hayhouse.com.au • *Published and distributed in the United Kingdom by:* Hay House UK, Ltd.: www.hayhouse.co.uk • *Published and distributed in the Republic of South Africa by:* Hay House SA (Pty), Ltd.: www.hayhouse.co.za • *Distributed in Canada by:* Raincoast Books: www.raincoast.com • *Published in India by:* Hay House Publishers India: www.hayhouse.co.in

Cover design: Michelle Polizzi
Book design: Tricia Breidenthal
Interior photos: Mitchell, Lisa, and Natalya Yass
Interior illustrations: Scott Leighton, Board Certified Medical Illustrator

Library of Congress Cataloging-in-Publication Data

Yass, Mitchell T, 1961-
  The pain cure Rx : the Yass method for diagnosing and resolving chronic pain / Dr. Mitchell Yass.
    pages cm
  ISBN 978-1-4019-4724-8 (hardback)
  1. Chronic pain--Treatment--Popular works. I. Title.
  RB127.Y37 2015
  616'.0472--dc23
                                2014044647

Hardcover ISBN: 978-1-4019-4724-8

10 9 8 7 6 5 4 3 2
1st edition, June 2015

Printed in the United States of America

To my wife, Lisa, who has seen
me through my darkest days,
and to my daughter, Natalya,
who is our light.

CONTENTS

INTRODUCTION

Chronic pain has become an international epidemic—an estimated one billion people across the globe suffer every day. And what I've found over my 20 years of treating pain is that many of these people suffer needlessly. While the existing medical model for treating pain isn't helping, there actually is hope—and that's what this book is about: an alternative model of treatment that resolves pain quickly and effectively without surgery or medication.

During my career, I have treated more than 14,000 patients, many of whom came to me as a last resort before surgery or as a follow-up after surgery that didn't resolve their pain. Many of them had been told that they would have to manage their pain using drugs for the rest of their lives or, worse, that there was nothing left to try in their efforts to find relief—they would simply have to live with the pain.

Case after case, I heard the same story: the patient had gone to the doctor, and diagnostic tests, like MRIs or X-rays, were done. A structural variation, such as a stenosis, a herniated disc, a meniscal tear, or arthritis, was found, and this became their diagnosis—it was the "cause" of their pain and they were treated based on this. Medications were used; injections, epidural nerve blocks, and a host of other treatments and procedures ensued. Some would mask the pain for a short time, but ultimately the pain returned and surgery was presented as the only remaining option. And then they had a terrible choice to make: get a surgery that didn't assure pain relief or try to manage the pain. In some cases patients were told that they would be paralyzed if surgery wasn't performed. Others were told that surgery may or may not help, and that it was in fact completely up to them when and if to move forward. In all cases, this horrible decision was left completely in the patient's hands.

The thousands of people who came to me were hoping for what they considered a miracle. What they didn't know was that there were no miracles needed. Resolving their pain was strictly a case of using logic and analysis to figure out the true cause of their pain, so it could be properly addressed.

In 90 to 95 percent of the cases where doctors had identified a structural problem as the cause of pain, I found something completely different. What I discovered as I worked with people was that most of the pain they experienced actually came from muscular weakness or imbalance rather than structural problems.

Let me explain how this works. People perform tasks every day: they walk, they move from sitting to standing, they climb stairs, they do all sorts of simple actions that require groups of muscles to work together. When one muscle is weak or out of commission because of an injury such as a strain, people still attempt to perform these tasks. However, to do this, the body must call on other muscles to compensate and work more than they are supposed to. This is what leads to muscle weakness or imbalance. The strained muscle can then emit pain or even cause a misalignment of joint surfaces that the muscles attach to, which can create pain at a joint.

I found that by looking at a person's symptoms rather than the findings from a diagnostic test, I was able to determine whether the cause of his or her pain was structural or muscular. The evidence became clear that the vast majority of patients had muscular causes. In these cases I was able to identify which muscles needed to be built up to resolve the weakness or imbalance causing the pain. And by having patients implement some simple exercises, I could help them overcome the pain they were feeling. Using this process, which I now refer to as the Yass Method, I wasn't providing minor pain relief; I was providing complete pain resolution.

This is what I want for you. As you work your way through the pages of this book, you will find the theoretical, clinical, and study-based evidence to understand why this process I have developed over 20 years works. This book will help you understand the true cause of your pain. By looking at things like your range of motion, flexibility, walking patterns, and posture, and combining this information with the interpretation of your symptoms, you will soon be able to identify if your pain is in fact muscular rather than structural. If it is structural, surgery is the proper course of action. However, if it is muscular, as a majority of the cases are, targeted strength training is the only answer.

I want to be emphatic about this point: If surgery is necessary, then all the exercise in the world will not resolve your pain. Conversely, if the cause of your pain is muscular, then all the surgeries in the world will not resolve your pain. If you've been treated by today's medical establishment, please do not simply believe that surgery is the last option—that everything else has been tried and surgery should be performed. This idea has led to an out-of-control rise in the number of people suffering from chronic pain. For those suffering from pain due to muscular causes, you have the power to treat your own pain naturally. And if you've already gone through surgery and still have pain, I hope this helps you see that there are safe and noninvasive ways to help yourself.

I believe it's time for a new paradigm of pain treatment to come to prominence. The evidence against the effectiveness of our current system grows every day. It's time to create a unified practice that is designed to understand the true cause of pain so we can provide the best possible treatment. Just like cardiology for the heart or dermatology for the skin, there needs to be one practice designed to address pain. Too many people's lives have been put on hold or destroyed. Too many people are hindered in what they can do. When walking up stairs or running after your child starts to become too difficult because of pain, your life changes in indescribable ways. It's not just a physical matter at that point; it's emotional. It's about quality of life and being able to do the things you love to do. Working solely within the confines of our current medical model, too many people have to contend with life-altering pain, but it doesn't have to be this way.

You can learn how to listen to your own body. You can learn how to look at your pain in a constructive and logical way. You have the power to help yourself. And who knows? Perhaps you can help spread the word that there is a path to a pain-free life. You've read about it. You've experienced it firsthand. And you're a shining example of success.

So sit back and enjoy the book—and then use the techniques. Soon you'll be back to your same old fully functioning self.

PART I

UNDERSTANDING
PAIN

CHAPTER 1

PAIN
TODAY

The statistics about chronic pain are staggering: one billion people across the globe, including an estimated 116 million American adults, suffer from this life-changing problem. But it doesn't just affect adults. I've treated people spanning in age from 6 to 96 years old. Nor does it target any particular type of person. It doesn't matter who you are or what you've accomplished in your life. It doesn't matter if you're an athlete or if you lead a sedentary life. Pain doesn't discriminate. We are all susceptible.

This is why chronic pain has become the number two reason people seek medical care—second only to symptoms associated with the common cold. In 2002, the cost of treating chronic pain was $70 billion. In 2011, the cost had ballooned to $635 billion. The total cost of health care was around $2.2 trillion. So if you think about it, $635 billion amounts to more than one-quarter of all healthcare costs—more than one dollar out of every four being spent went toward the treatment of chronic pain. To put this in perspective, in that same year, the estimated cost of treating cardiovascular disease was a little more than $400 billion.

The cost of this pain doesn't just apply to the individual; it goes much deeper, affecting the economy as a whole. The prevalence of pain has a tremendous impact on business, with a recent report by the Institute of Medicine indicating that the annual value of lost productivity in 2010 dollars ranged between $297.4 billion and $335.5 billion. The value of lost productivity is based on three estimates: days of work missed (ranging from $11.6 billion to $12.7 billion), hours of work lost (from $95.2 billion to $96.5 billion), and lower wages (from $190.6 billion to $226.3 billion). Compare this with a 2003 study published in the *Journal of the American Medical Association* that estimated the annual cost in lost productive time due to pain to be $61.2 billion, and you'll see that costs are just going up.

The rise in the cost of treating chronic pain has a direct effect on every person in the United States. These rising costs are part of what has led to our ever-increasing premiums and rise in deductibles from the insurance companies. Even if you have never suffered from chronic pain, you have been directly affected by the staggering rise in costs associated with treating it. The insurance companies use the same pool of premiums to pay for all medical treatments. If too many costs surpass premiums collected, three things occur: premiums must rise, copays and deductibles rise, and payments to practitioners decrease. I believe that treating chronic pain is one of the biggest reasons—if not *the* biggest reason—for the out-of-control health insurance industry for the past several years.

But aside from the financial costs, which are undeniable, I think the most devastating cost of pain is the physical and emotional impact it has on people's lives. People who come to my office are clearly suffering, and it's heartbreaking. They have been avoiding the things they love to do because it simply hurts too much. They have been leading lower-quality lives—sometimes for as much as 20 years. While it's true that I've treated patients who had no prior treatment before coming to see me, the majority of them have already been through the medical establishment. They've had multiple surgeries that did nothing to resolve their pain. They've taken drugs and had procedures that masked the pain, but they're still suffering. With this meteoric rise in money being spent on the treatment of chronic pain, why are more people today suffering for longer periods of time? What are we doing right now to deal with pain—and why isn't it working?

WHAT IS PAIN?

Before I jump into an explanation of how the current medical system looks at pain, I think it's important to understand what pain is. In its simplest form, pain is an attempt by the body to create a conscious awareness of bodily distress so that an intervention can be performed to resolve the distress. The U.S. Department of Health and Human Services' Agency for Healthcare Research and Quality defines pain as "an uncomfortable feeling that tells you something may be wrong in your body. Pain is your body's way of sending a warning to your brain." So pain is simply a notice from your body telling you that something needs to be taken care of.

To get a bit more technical: When the function of a tissue is compromised, the tissue sends a signal, which is identified by nociceptors (pain receptors). These nociceptors then send this information to the brain, which translates it into the sensation of pain.

One of the greatest misperceptions about pain is that it is solely associated with nerves. Most people who experience pain come to me thinking that the pain must be coming from a nerve and that to deal with the pain they have to deal with the nerve. However, this is simply not true. Pain receptors are found in their highest abundance in connective tissue, and connective tissue can be found in almost every tissue of every organ. This connective tissue typically sits around the cells of the organs, allowing for input regarding the health of the organ. If there is a breakdown in the cell of an organ, it sends a pain message to the brain.

So, yes, pain can be generated from the nerves; however, most tissues in the body have the ability to create these warning signals. Think about if you have pain from a kidney stone, a heart attack, an upset stomach, or a cut. It is the kidney, the heart, the stomach, or the skin that is releasing pain signals, sending them through pain receptors found in the connective tissue surrounding the cells that make up the tissues. Even muscles have the ability to send pain signals. In the example of the heart attack, the pain people experience is not because of a problem with the nerves. There is nothing wrong with the nerves; the pain is coming from the organ itself. The nerves are simply the pathway between the organ and the brain. The heart also often refers pain to the left arm—another pain that has nothing to do with the nerves.

There is a great paper written by Ginevra L. Liptan, M.D., that speaks directly to the power of pain receptors in connective tissue. Her focus was on pain receptors in the fascia of muscle as the cause of pain associated with fibromyalgia. She writes, "Central sensitization occurs when persistent nociceptive input leads to increased excitability in the dorsal horn neurons of the spinal cord. In this hyperexcited state, spinal cord neurons produce an enhanced responsiveness to noxious stimulation and even to formerly innocuous stimulation. . . . In fact, peripheral afferent nociceptors of muscle, the majority of which reside in the fascia, have been shown to be highly effective at causing central sensitization."[1] In plain English, what she is saying is that the pain of fibromyalgia can be attributed not to a nervous system dysfunction, but rather to an oversensitization of the pain receptors surrounding the muscle. Basically, any stimulation activates the pain sensors.

Sadly, the idea that all tissues can emit pain is something that hasn't been taken into account in our current pain treatment processes. If there is an obvious cause for the pain, such as a broken bone due to an accident or the pain associated with a heart attack, diagnosis is pretty simple. However, in the case of pain that is not attributable to a specific incident or tissue damage associated with an incident, the diagnostic tests used to identify the cause of pain focus mostly on structural abnormalities that might affect nerves. The primary mechanisms for identifying these structural issues are MRIs and X-rays. Using these techniques, doctors look for issues such as pinched nerves due to herniated discs or stenosis in the neck or back. Chronic pain that occurs anywhere in the body (especially in the limbs) is thought to be a "neuropathy"—structural damage to the nerves—stemming from the spine. This is also true if the symptoms experienced are tingling, burning, or numbness.

In reality, nonsystemic pain—pain that does not come from diseases, such as the pain associated with cancer, kidney stones, irritable bowel syndrome, and so on—can come from a number of different sources. It can be muscular, neurological, or structural. In our current pain treatment system, however, there is no one specialty that looks at all of these possibilities to determine which is correct—there is no one specialty capable of identifying which tissue is emitting the pain. There are about 15 different specialties that claim to understand the cause of pain and how to treat it—neurology, orthopedics, rheumatology, physiatry, podiatry, physical therapy, chiropractic, and acupuncture, just to name a few. But the practitioners in each of these fields are trained to see pain from their isolated educational and clinical experiences. Not one of these specialties is in a position to look at the big picture in order to identify the true cause of your pain.

Certainly most people understand that if you were to go to each one of these specialists to find the cause of your pain, you would most likely get several different and conflicting causes. As I like to say, "If you go to a surgeon, you'll likely need surgery." This is because surgeons are trained to look at a situation through the lens of how surgery can help. This is simply what they know. Don't get me wrong; this is not an indictment of the practitioners by any measure. This is an indictment of an educational system that allows pain to be a fringe issue that has not received its own specialty.

This splintered system of isolated specialists with partial understandings of pain, combined with the invalid methods of identifying the causes of pain, which are described in the next section, is the primary reason our current medical system has been ineffective at dealing with pain.

Luckily, this is beginning to change.

CHANGING PERSPECTIVES

While a unified specialty that looks at all possible causes of pain has not yet taken hold, people are beginning to see the flaws in our current system. In February 2011, in a stunning position paper, the American College of Physicians recommended that MRIs no longer be used to identify the cause of pain at the lower back. It noted that in 85 percent of patients with lower back pain, their pain could not be attributed to a spinal abnormality like a herniated disc, stenosis, or a disease. The causes were deemed "nonspecific." The paper went on to note that tests like these lead to unnecessary treatments and procedures and simply increase costs. It was also noted that the identification of structural abnormalities with complex medical terms that are unknown to the layperson leads to unnecessary stress for patients. The relevance of this finding cannot be overlooked or discarded.

I have found that, in cases where people are diagnosed with something, they end up focusing solely on the medical phrases because they seem so ominous. This can be a problem, because when people focus on the fear-inducing terminology more than the meaning of the words, they begin to believe that something has gone very wrong for them and thus opt for unnecessarily intense treatments. A great example of this is the diagnosis of stenosis of the spine. While this sounds horrible, the word *stenosis* simply means narrowing. The patient may have extremely mild stenosis, which is not actually causing any symptoms, and yet he or she can be talked into getting surgery or other unnecessary treatments because the word sounds so dangerous.

A great number of studies led up to the position paper by the American College of Physicians. This area of study has, in fact, been growing immensely in the past few decades. The first study that showed a conflict between positive MRI findings and a correlation to pain occurred all the way back in 1994. The study showed that roughly 70 percent of people with absolutely no pain had either bulging or herniated discs.

The 2008 article "The Pain May Be Real, but the Scan Is Deceiving," by Gina Kolata, which was published in *The New York Times,* focused on similar findings. It picked up on the idea that MRIs find structural abnormalities in as many people with no pain as in those with pain, thus leading to the conclusion that these abnormalities are not the cause of pain. The article quotes Dr. David Felson, a professor of medicine and epidemiology at Boston University Medical School, saying,

"Every time we get a new technology that provides insights into structures we didn't encounter before, we end up saying, 'Oh, my God, look at all those abnormalities.' They might be dangerous . . . Some are, some aren't, but it ends up leading to a lot of care that's unnecessary."

The research of David Felson went a bit deeper into this phenomenon. In a study published in the September 2011 issue of *The New England Journal of Medicine,* Dr. Felson's team found that meniscal tears were just as common in people with knee arthritis who did not complain of pain as they were in people with knee arthritis who did have pain. They tended to occur along with arthritis and were a part of the degenerative process itself. This means that repairing the tears would not eliminate the pain.

Dr. James Andrews, a widely known sports medicine orthopedist in Gulf Breeze, Florida, wanted to test his suspicions that MRIs, which are given to almost every injured athlete or casual exerciser, might be a bit misleading. So he scanned the shoulders of 31 perfectly healthy professional baseball pitchers.

The pitchers were not injured and had no pain. But the MRIs found abnormal shoulder cartilage in 90 percent of them and abnormal rotator cuff tendons in 87 percent. "If you want an excuse to operate on a pitcher's throwing shoulder, just get an MRI," Dr. Andrews says.[2]

To look at this premise of the MRI not finding the cause of pain from another angle, we can consider studies and statistics of surgical procedures performed on these diagnosed structural abnormalities.

In 2002, *The New England Journal of Medicine* highlighted a study that attempted to link the surgical removal of arthritis from the knee with the resolution of knee pain. All the patients in the study had been diagnosed with arthritis as the cause of the knee pain. These people were divided into three groups: one group received an arthroscopic debridement in which the arthritic tissue was surgically removed, one group received an arthroscopic lavage in which the joint was washed (rinsed), and one group had a placebo surgery. Neither the patients nor assessors were told which group the people had been assigned to. What they found was that there was no discernable difference between the results of the actual procedures and the placebo procedure. The conclusion of the study was clear and concise: "In patients with osteoarthritis of the knee, arthroscopic surgery did not relieve pain or improve function more than a placebo procedure."[3]

What I want people to understand about these findings is what the placebo group means. When people in the placebo group improve, the change is simply due to a belief that they are getting treatment and thus will feel better. In this case, those in the placebo group who felt a reduction in pain simply felt the decreased pain because they believed they would. To fully understand the true effectiveness of a procedure, you must discount the same number of people who felt improvement in the placebo group from the group who had the actual procedure, because you have to assume a similar number improved solely as a result of belief. In this case, since the findings were exactly the same between a real surgery and a placebo, this indicates that surgery did not play a role in improving pain. It is a stunning testament to the fact that the arthritis could not have been the cause of the knee pain.

While the studies about placebos are interesting, to me one of the biggest indications that surgery based solely on a diagnosis of a structural variation is problematic came with the introduction of the term *failed back surgery syndrome.* Several years ago, the rate of failure from neck and spine surgery rose so high that the medical establishment was forced to coin a phrase for those who still had the same if not greater pain at the neck or back after the surgery.

We can see just how terrible the results of back surgery have been. In a study presented in the medical journal *Spine,* it was determined that spinal fusion failed in 74 percent of cases of workers' compensation subjects. Of the group that received spinal fusions for lower back pain, only 26 percent of them returned to work versus 67 percent of those who did not have surgery. This is a staggering number. The reoperation rate for those who had surgery was 27 percent. Of those who had lumbar fusion, 36 percent had complications. And permanent disability rates were 11 percent for the population who had surgery versus just 2 percent for the nonsurgical population.

Thank goodness, many major medical bodies now agree with the premise that herniated discs found on MRIs do not necessarily represent the cause of lower back pain. The *Arthritis Advisor* for July 2011 from the Cleveland Clinic noted, "Most back pain is muscular." The article goes on to say, "What has given spine surgery a bad name is people having fusions for back pain when there is no instability. They get an MRI because of the pain; it shows an abnormal disk and so they get a fusion. That's a terrible indication because you don't know that the disk is the source of the pain. Disk degeneration is a normal phenomenon of aging; everybody eventually suffers from it."[4]

The fact is you don't have to look at medical journals for studies or medical bodies to confirm that something is wrong with the way pain is addressed in the existing medical model. Look at yourself, your family members, and your friends and see how many of them are being treated for pain through the use of pain management. This practice is so out of control it has led to the need for state regulations to restrict its use. And if you think about it, the idea of managing pain seems bizarre and medieval. Medical care should focus on eliminating pain, not simply managing it. If pain is an indication that something has gone wrong in the body, the goal should be to identify the tissue emitting the pain signal and resolve the distress of the tissue. This ends the need for a pain signal and it ceases. Clearly the existing model doesn't work.

BRINGING IT ALL BACK

I know I've laid out a lot of evidence showing that our current medical system is failing, but I've found that when I work with people, these explanations don't necessarily put everything in perspective. They don't help most people understand what's causing pain and why our system doesn't address it well. So let me put this in terms that we can all understand. It's a metaphor that I use all the time: your body as a car.

Let's say there is a car parked on the street. For some reason, I decide to take a sledgehammer and beat the hell out of the driver's door panel. Then I let the air out of all four tires. After doing this damage, I get in the car and start it up. I put it in drive, but the car won't move.

As I try to figure out why it is stranded in place, I call in a friend. My friend looks at the car and then looks at me and says, "It's obvious what's wrong. You have a bashed-in driver's door panel. Anybody can see that. I can take a picture of it. I can show you the picture and prove that the door is bashed in."

But that just doesn't make sense. Cars can still go when they have a ruined door. This doesn't affect their mechanics. So in this instance, what should have been noted is that the car is running and in drive; it's just not moving. This would imply that the flat tires are actually the problem. Fill up the tires and you'll be good to go. Yes, the structure of the car has been damaged, but the door is not causing the problem. The bashed-in door panel in this example represents the herniated disc, stenosis, arthritis, or meniscal tear that doctors find on MRIs. Just as with the door panel, just because the structural problem can be found doesn't mean it is the cause of the symptom. *Understanding the symptom is the key to understanding the cause.*

Looking simply at the door is the equivalent of looking simply at structural deficiencies in the body. I have unfortunately treated way too many people after they had the "door panel" surgically repaired only to find that their car still wasn't moving correctly. It just doesn't make sense. So what's the answer?

CHAPTER 2

A NEW MODEL OF **PAIN DIAGNOSIS** AND **RESOLUTION**

I hope we can all agree that a banged-up door doesn't strand a car in one place. The car not moving is a symptom, and that's what we have to look at to figure out what's gone wrong. I don't know any good mechanic who would claim, in this instance, that the door was the problem. They would see that the car couldn't move, and they would focus straight in on the tires. When you think about diagnosis in this way, it seems absurd that the current medical system looks solely at the physical equivalent of the door.

And that's what makes the Yass Method different. It looks at the overall situation, not simply the structural issues. But before I jump into the specifics of my process, let's go back to the car metaphor for a moment. Let's say the car—the one with the ruined driver's door panel—is sitting in the street. You get into the car and put the key in the ignition, but the motor won't turn over. Again, in this situation, it should be obvious that the problem isn't the door. In this case, the likely problem is that the battery is dead. There is a clear correlation between the symptom (the car not starting) and the cause (the battery being dead). It's not the door!

I'm not saying that a bashed-in door couldn't cause problems. But if you think logically about it, a bashed-in door would only cause door-related problems. If you can't get into the car because the door won't open, that's likely due to the damaged door panel.

Only in this last situation do the symptoms indicate that the cause was the damage to the door. In the prior two cases, you could spend thousands of dollars to replace the door panel, and you would still face the same problem—either your car won't move because of the tires or the engine won't turn over because of the battery.

The same is true with your body. Your herniated disc, your arthritis, your meniscal tear—your very own bashed-in door—isn't necessarily the cause of your pain. Let's jump back for a moment to that first study we discussed that showed a conflict between positive MRI findings and a correlation to pain. In this study, presented in *The New England Journal of Medicine,* researchers decided to perform MRIs on people who were in no pain at all. The tests showed that roughly 70 percent of these people had either bulging or herniated discs. The significance of the finding is astounding! Think about it. If roughly 70 percent of people with no pain have bulging or herniated discs, then it can be extrapolated that in roughly 70 percent of people with pain *and* a bulging or herniated disc, the pain is coming from another source. I couldn't have stated it any better than the authors of the study in their conclusion: "On MRI examination of the lumbar spine, many people without back pain have disk bulges or protrusions but not extrusions. Given the high prevalence of these findings and of back pain, the discovery by MRI of bulges or protrusions in people with low back pain may frequently be coincidental."[5]

As I mentioned before, I've found that about 90 percent of the people I work with have been misdiagnosed using the current medical model. Ninety percent! That's crazy. I've had patients who were rushed to the hospital because of intense pain in the gluteal (buttocks) region and were diagnosed with stenosis after an MRI was taken. I saw them after they left the hospital and, using the Yass Method, was able to identify the cause of the pain as a muscle spasm—nothing more. With a couple of treatments, the pain was resolved and the patient's ability to move and function was fully restored.

By looking at the symptoms along with the outcome of some simple tests, which I describe in the next chapter, I am able to put together a full picture of what's gone wrong. While structural abnormalities *can* cause pain, we can only definitively know that this is the cause if we determine some other things first. And most of the time, I find that the pain is coming from a muscular imbalance or weakness rather than a structural abnormality.

So for every patient I see, I start by ignoring any diagnostic test findings. Instead, I ask them questions about their ability to move around. About where the pain is being experienced. About what makes that pain worse or better. And about whether there was a specific incident that brought on the symptom.

Then I use this information, along with the data I get from simple clinical tests that look at range of motion, flexibility, functional testing, and posture, to understand the true source of pain. If my evaluation suggests that the cause of the pain is structural, then I fully endorse the use of a diagnostic test like an MRI or X-ray to confirm my finding. If my evaluation yields a finding that the cause of the pain is muscle weakness or imbalance, then all the diagnostic tests in the world will do nothing to further the resolution of the symptoms. The key is to let the interpretation of the symptoms be the guide to identifying the cause of the symptoms.

If the problem is muscular-based, there's so much more you can do on your own—without surgery or medication. And I'll walk you through all of it in the second half of this book.

BEGINNING THE JOURNEY

The beginning of this symptom-focused method began for me when I entered medical school at the ripe old age of 30. In my 20s, I was actually a project manager in interior contracting, a difficult position that forced me to take on a lot of responsibility while being completely dependent on others—carpenters, plumbers, electricians, and various other subcontractors—to complete the work. Ultimately, the stress of this job got the best of me, and I decided I needed a new direction. So for six weeks I simply contemplated what I could do for the rest of my life.

Other than construction, the only thing I really did actively was weight lifting. I had been lifting for a couple of years and really enjoyed how it made me feel, so I left the construction business and took a job in a gym cleaning up and helping people with their weight-lifting technique. The very first guy I met had a master's degree in exercise physiology, and he turned me on to the idea of occupational therapy, athletic training, and physical therapy. Each of these areas worked with the body and muscle systems, so they all interested me, but in the end, physical therapy seemed like the best fit since it got most deeply into the nuts and bolts of the human body and the interrelationship of the tissues of the body.

I note these things only because I think it is important to understand my state of mind when I began my physical therapy studies. I had a lot of experience from my career in construction, and I had learned some hard lessons about life. This means that I knew how to handle the pressure of medical school—in fact, after the work I'd done, this pressure felt, well, like very little pressure at all! I was no longer in charge of millions of dollars of contracts. I didn't have to try to control other people. I wasn't interacting with businesses that had put millions of dollars on the line. I think this is what made me different from the other students, most of whom were very young, with little life experience to help them deal with the pressures of medical school or the need for critical thought. They were feverishly trying to memorize every single thing that was placed in front of them—because this is simply what they had always done. They didn't stop and think, but my experience helped me understand that every situation is unique. While you do have to know the facts of a situation and understand the elements that are true throughout, it is even more important to be able to use critical thinking and logic when looking at each particular situation to see what varies. Because I understood this, my goal for medical school was to learn the important things (and enough to pass my tests) and leave myself open for analyzing what was put before me. This freed up my mind tremendously.

The other quality I had that gave me a different viewpoint than other students was that throughout my life, my father, an electronics engineer with his college degree in physics who designed intercom systems for the country's most significant weapon systems, had stressed the importance of analytical thinking. When I was about nine, I decided that I wanted to be just like my father and began to understand how to think like him. He was adamant about the fact that logic was king. It didn't matter if something was spoken or written; if it didn't pass the test of logical analysis, it could not be accepted as fact. While growing up, I thought my father was the smartest person in the world, and so I clung to every word he spoke. I took his theories about proof to heart, and through my teen years I developed my ability to analyze information for validity. I did not accept anything as a fact unless it was logical.

These two factors set the stage for my medical school experience and for the development of the Yass Method.

QUESTIONS BEING RAISED

As school progressed, I started to question some of the material being taught. One of the first big conflicts came when the subject of traction was discussed. We were taught about traction, in which a device uses a mechanical pulling force to separate the vertebrae to take pressure off a herniated disc and thus resolve any pain coming from the disc. We were taught that for lumbar (lower back) traction to be successful, it would require half the person's body weight in pressure to achieve enough separation. So for a guy who weighed 225 pounds, it would take about 110 pounds of pressure to provide relief. Makes sense. However, when we got instruction on using the traction machine, I was told that you typically never use more than about 40 to 50 pounds of pressure. Most of the other students simply accepted this idea—either because they were really excited by this cool machine or because of their acceptance of the "experts" who were teaching. But for me, there was something just not right about this situation. If someone needs 110 pounds of pressure to separate the vertebrae enough to take pressure off a disc to resolve pain, why is the standard only 40 to 50 pounds? This just didn't compute. And it forced me to think about the whole treatment and its purpose.

I was being told that this modality was designed to separate the vertebrae so pressure could be taken off intervertebral discs. In anatomy class, I had learned that there are five ligaments designed to keep the vertebrae in alignment to protect the spinal cord. Did it really make sense, with this natural form of protection in place, that vertebral discs should be separated by an external force? Then I began to think about the mechanism itself. The traction system works by placing belts around the rib cage and at the top of the pelvis. If you wanted to create the resistance necessary to separate the vertebrae, could this mechanism achieve the goal? The answer is an absolute no. The belts would create so much friction against the ribs and pelvis that it would be too painful. Also, the belts would most likely slide, preventing enough tension from being developed. Ultimately the only logical conclusion I could come to as to why this was bringing lower back relief was that this technique was simply stretching the lower back muscles—nothing more. I couldn't believe that this was being taught as a way to separate vertebrae when it seemed impossible that this was the case.

Another issue that concerned me was using electrical stimulation to treat pain. We were taught that the sensation of pain and the sensation of touch experienced at the skin enter the brain at the same location. The one that is experienced with the highest intensity is the one that the brain identifies. So if you increase the sensation of touch, then pain will not be experienced. By causing skin in an area where pain was being experienced to instead feel the sensory stimulation created by an electrical surge, you will no longer experience the pain. I immediately thought, *Well, this is good for a short-term concept, but what happens when the electrical stimulation ends? What is going to stop the pain from returning?*

Then there were the big philosophical questions that arose. I was being taught that techniques like electrical stimulation, ultrasound, and massage would address the supposed causes of pain, such as herniated discs, arthritis, and stenosis. I could in no way accept this. How on earth did any of these things change the body structurally? I was extremely confused. The treatment modalities I was learning seemed to have no logical basis. This lack of treating structural abnormalities even seemed to be recognized in the physical therapy profession itself. Physical therapy is considered palliative care, which means that it is never intended to resolve the cause of pain, simply to diminish the effects.

Things really became questionable when I started performing my affiliations, the equivalent of a residency for a physician—a time during which you treat patients under the supervision of a clinical instructor. I was treating patients based on diagnoses, but the diagnoses didn't seem to match the symptoms the patients described. One early case that sticks out in my memory was a patient who came in with a diagnosis of pain due to a meniscal tear of the knee. This basically means that the cartilage of his knee joint was torn. In school, we had learned that the pain expected from a meniscal tear would be at the joint line (space between the thigh bone and lower leg bone) at either side of the knee. However, when I asked the patient to point to exactly where he was experiencing pain, he pointed to an area around his kneecap. When I tried to press on the spot he was complaining about, I was pressing on the sides of his kneecap. This was extremely confusing, because if the meniscus was the cause of pain, it could never create pain at that location.

This happened with patient after patient who came in with a meniscal tear. For some, it would be pain around the kneecap. For others, it would be where the hamstring (posterior thigh muscle) tendon attaches just below the knee joint. And this didn't happen just with meniscal tears. I found similar inconsistencies when I saw patients who had been diagnosed with arthritis, herniated discs, and all sorts of other structural abnormalities.

Another confusion I faced was that many of the patients I saw lacked other symptoms that are expected with these diagnoses. The issue that brought this most to light for me was that very few patients were experiencing a loss in range of motion. If the cause of their pain was a structural abnormality that compromised the integrity of the joint, they should be experiencing a loss in range of motion along with their pain. Since a joint is nothing more than a pivot point where two bones come together, a variation to the structure of the joint should change how those two bones interact. For example, if your knee joint is compromised, this should result in an inability to bend or straighten the knee like normal. This loss in range of motion should happen whether you try to move your knee or you have someone else try to move it for you.

The next thing that upped my confusion was the treatment being provided for arthritis, which is one of the most common diagnoses given for pain at peripheral joints like the shoulders, wrists, hands, hips, knees, and ankles. The primary method for treating the arthritis was either a cortisone shot or some form of anti-inflammatory drug. But osteoarthritis is not an inflammatory disease; it's a mechanical wearing away of joint surfaces. Also, with most of these patients, there was never an indication that an inflammatory response was occurring. If it were, they would experience not only pain but also heat and swelling. Look at other situations where an inflammatory response is clearly occurring: a sprained ankle, a contusion, a pimple, the flu. In every one of these cases, the three key ingredients that indicate an inflammatory response exist. So with the arthritis diagnosis, not only are you getting a treatment that doesn't match the key characteristics of the condition, you are also getting treatment that doesn't match the symptoms. The treatment is based on the idea that pain equals inflammation. But as you can see from things such as a heart attack or kidney stones or even something as simple as a pinch, you can have pain without inflammation. Let's be clear; if pain is due to an inflammatory response, then the use of anti-inflammatory drugs and treatments makes sense. But if the cause of pain is unrelated to an inflammatory response, as is the case with arthritis, the use of anti-inflammatory drugs is of no value and will do nothing to resolve the cause of the pain.

The other big red flag for me was that in most cases, patients couldn't remember a specific incident that caused their symptoms. Tearing of cartilage in the knee, for example, doesn't just happen—generally this comes from a traumatic event, such as overextension, excessively bending the knee, or twisting the knee. Most people told me they didn't remember when their pain began. Whatever the case, it was rarely associated with trauma. Also, the vast majority of patients never mentioned noticing swelling or bleeding that would be expected with an injury. The association between a structural abnormality caused by a traumatic event and just a degenerative structural abnormality confused a lot of people. For those who experienced a traumatic event that led to a structural variation, the onset of pain would be associated with that event. But the types of structural variations found on diagnostic tests are for the most part chronic in nature. They are progressive and develop so slowly that they do not even ignite a pain signal. This is how you account for the roughly 70 percent of people with structural variations but no pain found in that first 1994 study. Simply finding structural variations, such as a torn meniscus or rotator cuff, is meaningless in regard to pain unless they are also associated with a traumatic event. In this case, there is a much higher likelihood that the structural variation is the cause of pain.

For almost every patient I saw and at almost every part of the body, diagnoses were popping up that didn't make sense. The diagnosed cause could not create the symptoms being experienced. And the more time I spent looking at the diagnoses being given and the symptoms being experienced, the more I began to realize that the diagnoses were flawed. The structural variations being identified had nothing to do with the cause of the symptoms. But at this point, I wasn't sure what the true cause could be.

DEVELOPING MY METHOD

I finally graduated from physical therapy school and landed my first job working for a physical therapist. He was out of the office a lot because of other business responsibilities, which meant that I was on my own most of the time. I was a fresh graduate left alone to diagnose and treat patients with virtually no supervision. Because of the questionable information I was given in physical therapy school, the concerns I had developed during my affiliations, and the initial studies that were now coming out against using MRIs and other diagnostic tests to find the cause of pain, I felt certain that standard pain-treatment procedures were not the answer.

However, coming out of school I didn't feel comfortable that I truly understood what pain was or what was causing it. All I knew was that the current practices were wrong. I felt that if I was going to treat pain, I needed a complete understanding as to why it exists and how it is transmitted. So I began to think about pain that comes in other situations.

If a person eats bad fish and has severe stomach pain, they don't get an MRI to determine the origin of the pain, nor are they referred to a neurologist. The pain is accepted as a signal from the stomach lining that something in the stomach shouldn't be there. That's it. Once the bad fish is passed or expelled, the pain signal is no longer necessary and the stomach pain ceases. If somebody has a cut, the same premise works. Once the cut is treated, the pain simply ends. I decided to think of resolving pain at the neck, back, or peripheral joints in the same way: I needed to identify which tissue was creating the pain signal and address the distress of that tissue.

As I worked with more and more patients, I started to notice that most of them associated their pain with functional tasks, like climbing stairs or getting out of a car. They sometimes associated their pain with recreational activities, like playing golf or tennis. And many of them associated their pain with performing work-related activities. Almost everyone said that they were not in pain when they were doing nothing. This really hit home to me as a logician. I recognized that function results from muscles working together. Since the pain seemed to mostly be associated with specific functional tasks, this directed me to certain muscles that might be in distress and thus were sending pain signals.

Because of this, I felt I needed to understand more about what was happening with the muscle. Why was it straining and thus emitting pain? What was preventing it from performing certain functional tasks? I had a general sense that the muscle must not have enough strength to perform the task and this triggered the muscle to strain, but I needed to understand more.

The theory I began to develop was based on the success I had when I treated muscles to resolve the pain and allow normal function to return. This treatment had been focused on knots in the muscle. What I saw was that when muscle strained, knots developed. I could press on these knots and they would incite the same pain the patient was complaining of. I also saw that the muscle had a loss of strength and flexibility due to the knots. On the basis of this experience, I came up with a theory to explain the presence of the knots before treatment and the fact that they weren't there after treatment.

There is fluid in muscle that provides lubrication that allows the muscle to create force. When a muscle is required to create more force than it is naturally capable of because of the demand of a task, the body sees this as dangerous—something that could potentially cause the muscle to tear. To prevent this from occurring, the body converts the water-based fluid to a thicker, gluey substance that has the capacity to bind muscle fiber together. This prevents the muscle from tearing, but it also prevents it from being able to reach its normal length. This, in turn, means that it cannot create its maximal force, which eventually leads to it straining if it continues to be required to perform a difficult functional task. The gluing together of the muscle fibers also causes the pain receptors that surround them to become more concentrated. This increased concentration of pain receptors is the reason the knots are so painful to the touch. Breaking up the knots, I found, achieves three immediate goals: it increases range of motion of the muscle, it increases strength of the muscle, and it decreases pain in the muscle. This theory of a change in consistency of the muscle fluid is strictly mine, and it explains the experiences I have had in treating muscle in order to change its ability to perform functional tasks while decreasing symptoms.

Since there was such overwhelming evidence from the experiences I was having clinically, including the success of treating muscles, and the studies I was reading, I developed a new thought process. I began to associate joint pain with the forces on joints rather than the joint's structure itself.

This began my intense study of how our muscles work together and how an imbalance or weakness in one muscle could create pain. I looked at the muscle systems and associated physical structures like a machine—one part affects another and then that part affects another and so on. So, for instance, the primary group of muscles and physical structures that work together to perform most weight-bearing activities, such as walking or jogging, include:

- Quadriceps muscle
- Quad tendon
- Patella (kneecap)
- Patella tendon
- Tibial tuberosity (a projection on the lower leg bone where the patella tendon attaches)

A strain of the quadriceps muscle could produce a variety of symptoms, including pain at the front of the thigh, around the kneecap, at the quad or patella tendon, or even the tibial tuberosity. A strained quad could also cause irritation around the kneecap—enough to create swelling (synovitis) in the joint. It could also affect the body's ability to bring fluid from the extremities through the lymphatic system, which would cause swelling in the lower leg. So what you see are myriad symptoms that can be potentially attributed to the same cause: a strained quad. The key to my understanding was that regardless of where the symptoms manifested, ultimately the only way to resolve the symptoms was to strengthen the quad muscles.

Understanding these systems inside and out became the goal of my practice. If these systems were clearly mapped out, I could use logical analysis to help me figure out the true cause of people's pain—it would allow me to figure out which tissue was in distress and emitting the pain signal.

FLESHING OUT MY METHOD

I began to use clinical tests, such as functional testing, to guide my decision making. For example, I would have a patient complaining of gluteal (buttocks) pain try to perform certain functional tasks like standing on one foot, squatting, or hopping to see which task brought on the pain. If they had difficulty standing on one leg, it would tell me that the gluteus medius—the hip muscle associated with balance—was weak. Since the gluteus medius and piriformis (another muscle found in the gluteal region) work together to create balance, I could then examine these two muscles to see whether the distressed tissue was the gluteus medius itself or the piriformis. Using palpation and flexibility testing, I could see which muscle was emitting pain or if it was severely shortened because of straining. I will go much further into how clinical tests allow me to differentiate the cause of pain in the next chapter.

One idea that helped me develop my process was the use of tests that differentiate between referred pain and point-tender pain. By definition, *referred pain* describes pain that is experienced in one location while the cause of the pain is at another location. *Point-tender pain* is defined as pain that is experienced in the same location as the tissue that is emitting the pain signal. This differentiation is essential to diagnosing which tissue is emitting the pain signal.

Let's look at a patient with pain across the whole lower back. If this pain were being caused by a herniated disc in the lumbar spine, the implication would be that the pain was being referred from the lumbar spine. Logically, then, if you wanted to increase the pain, you would have to press on the lumbar spine. If you were to press at the lower back region away from the spine, there should be no alteration in the intensity of the pain. When I pressed on the lower back away from the spine—in the spot where the pain was being experienced—and my patient jumped in pain, I understood that they were experiencing point-tender pain rather than referred pain, which meant that the pain couldn't be from the lumbar spine. It had to be coming from the tissue I was pressing on.

Pain referral does not just stop there. It's not a choice of the pain coming simply from one or the other—referred from the structural abnormality or the muscle emitting the symptom. What I recognized is that pain can be referred by muscles, not just nerves—an idea that isn't very popular in the medical community. For the most part, what is accepted is that pain can only be referred from the spine. Pain or an altered sensation at the hand or foot, for example, immediately leads to an MRI of the cervical or lumbar spine. However, over 20 years of working with patients, I've found that this simply isn't true. For example, one of the primary causes of pain or altered sensation in the hand is a referred symptom from the rotator cuff or shoulder blade stabilizing muscles. I could press on the muscle at the shoulder or shoulder blade and it would bring on the symptom in the hand. Many of the patients in whom I found this had been told that the problem in their hand was due to a herniated disc or stenosis in the cervical spine. I'm not sure why pain referred by muscle isn't accepted or more commonly acknowledged for chronic pain, because it is acknowledged in cases of acute pain. Think about when someone is having a heart attack. A potential indicator is pain in their left arm. Clearly, there is nothing wrong with their arm. The pain being experienced is referred from the heart, which happens to be a muscle.

Another mechanism that seems to lack any acknowledgment as a potential cause of pain is the idea of a strained muscle impinging on a nerve. In a study led by William Ryan, he identifies that the common peroneal nerve can be impinged at the "fibular tunnel," which is basically a tunnel-like opening where two muscles—the soleus and the peroneus longus—converge. In an instance like this, one of these converging muscles can strain and thicken, and, because of its close proximity to a nerve, it can impinge on a nerve or group of nerves referring symptoms to another location. This is precisely what happens in carpal tunnel syndrome. The median nerve is compressed by the finger and wrist flexor tendons as it runs through the carpal tunnel. While nerve impingement is accepted as the cause of carpal tunnel syndrome, it is not given as the cause of sciatica, which is possibly the greatest example of this phenomenon. In fact, in almost every case of sciatica (pain that ranges from the gluteal region to the foot), the cause is a strained piriformis muscle impinging on the sciatic nerve in the gluteal region, a fact that was confirmed by Aaron Filler by use of the MRN (magnetic resonance neurography). In his studies, 93 percent of cases of sciatica were due to this type of muscular impingement of a nerve.

Whether the cause of the symptom is a strained muscle, a strained muscle referring a symptom, or a strained muscle impinging on a nerve, ultimately the use of diagnostic tests cannot identify these potential causes. Misdiagnosis is almost guaranteed, which is why these three causes account for more than 90 percent of cases I have treated. The most effective method I have found, which is the underpinning to diagnosis in the Yass Method, is to use clinical tests to determine a cause. This analysis must include a clear understanding of a possible mechanism of injury, the type and intensity of the symptoms, and the location of the symptoms. Is the symptom point-tender or is it referred? If it is referred, what are the possible mechanisms for referring the symptom? Is it possible that the symptom is referred from a muscle or is it referred by a strained muscle that is impinging on a nerve?

If these types of questions have not been a part of your evaluation, I believe that a thorough attempt to understand the cause of your symptoms has not been made. There is absolutely nothing more important than achieving a successful diagnosis, because an incorrect diagnosis leads to incorrect treatment. A proper diagnosis means treatment can be performed accurately with very specific intentions to resolve a cause.

CHAPTER 3

TESTING
PROCEDURES

Now that you have a general understanding of what's involved in the Yass Method—the philosophy and general practices—I want to delve more deeply into the clinical tests that help me find the true causes of my patients' pain. This chapter explains in detail the specifics of the individual techniques so you can begin to incorporate them into an understanding of how to get a proper diagnosis of your symptoms. The key is to learn not only how to perform the tests but also how to organize the findings into a coherent narrative of what's causing your pain.

Clinical evaluation should be seen as a tool designed to tell a story. Each technique I talk about below should not be used individually—the information you gather builds on itself with one test confirming the outcome of another. Once all the tests are performed, you should be able to develop a complete narrative that explains what tissue is causing the pain, what caused the tissue to break down, what the clinical indicators are that explain this theory, and what can be done to resolve the cause of the pain.

One note: please do not attempt to use any of these tests as you're reading this chapter. These descriptions cover only why the tests are important and what you can learn from them. I will give detailed instructions about how to do each of these tests in the second half of the book.

TECHNIQUE 1: RANGE-OF-MOTION TEST

The range-of-motion test is probably the most significant test to understand when determining if the cause of pain is a structural abnormality, such as arthritis or a meniscal tear, or if the pain is due to muscular problems, from a condition such as a muscle strain or imbalance. This technique looks at what type of available range of motion exists at the joint where you feel pain.

Before we talk about the test itself, it's important to understand that joints are composed of two bones coming together with a space between them. This space is usually filled with cartilage that maintains a gap between the bones as they move. The joint should be perceived as nothing more than a pivot point: a place where movement can develop to allow the limbs to perform functional activities. The joint is stabilized and moved by the muscles that pass by it. There are two general reasons why a joint may not be able to move through its full range of motion:

1. There is some change in the structural integrity of the joint. This occurs when the joint space between the bones is compromised. This leads to a structural inhibition of motion.

2. The muscles situating the bones in the joint are strained or imbalanced. If there is a muscle weakness or imbalance, the bone surfaces that make up the joint can become misaligned, causing abnormal rubbing that can lead to pain that leads to lost range of motion.

This distinction becomes important when you look at range of motion because there are two types of range of motion: active and passive. *Active* range of motion refers to how far you can move your joint on your own. *Passive* refers to how far someone else can move your joint. The relationship between how much a joint can be moved actively versus passively will help you identify whether the cause of pain is structural or muscular. The use of this test pertains to joints like the shoulder, hip, and knee.

When looking at the range of motion that is available at a particular joint, you are not trying to identify the exact range of motion. What you are interested in is whether the active and passive ranges of motion are the same or different. You are also looking at the range of motion in relation to a similar joint that is not experiencing pain. So, for example, you would compare your painful left knee with your pain-free right knee. After doing these tests, there are only two options:

Option 1: If passive range of motion and active range of motion are the same *and* this range of motion is less than a similar joint, then the problem is structural.

Option 2: If the passive range of motion is greater than the active range of motion *and* it is similar to or mildly less than the range of motion of a similar joint, then the problem is not structural.

Let's look at the knee example again to make this more clear. To get information from the range-of-motion test, you would:

1. Move your painful left knee on your own and look at how far you are able to move it.

2. Have someone else move your painful left knee and look at how far they can move it.

3. Ask yourself if the outcomes are the same or different.

4. Have someone else move your pain-free right knee and look at how far it can move.

5. Ask yourself if this is more than the range of the left knee.

If step 1 and step 2 are the same, this implies that there is a structural problem. This range of motion should also be decreased in comparison to the other similar joint.

If the cause of pain is muscular, then the active range of motion is decreased; however, the passive range of motion is almost if not completely full in comparison to the side with no pain.

This is a critical point to understand. I have had thousands of cases where a patient was told that the cause of their joint pain was due to arthritis, a labral tear, or a meniscal tear based simply on an MRI or X-ray finding. I'm not saying that these structural variations didn't exist. The question is to what degree did they exist? If the variation was small enough to not cause a change in the integrity of the joint, then the joint will work perfectly even with the variation. The way to determine whether these findings are causing the pain is to look at the function of the joint. In almost every one of the cases where a structural variation was diagnosed as the cause of pain, I found that the joint went through almost complete, if not fully complete, range of motion. This told me that the structure of the joint was intact and that the finding had nothing to do with the patient's pain. Once this was established, I would move on to the next test in my arsenal: muscle testing.

TECHNIQUE 2: MUSCLE TESTING

The use of muscle testing is not necessarily an attempt to create a quantifiable level of strength of a muscle or group of muscles. In the Yass Method it is used to help confirm a diagnosis. For instance, when a person has an MRI showing a torn meniscus (cartilage), muscle testing can help me determine if their pain is from the tear or from the muscles that surround the knee, such as the hamstrings (posterior thigh muscle) and quadriceps (front thigh muscle). In a quick muscle test, I should be able to see if there is a difference in strength between the painful knee and the pain-free knee and if the pain increases during the test. Just as with the range-of-motion test, there are two basic outcomes in this test:

Option 1: There is no difference in strength between the knee with pain and the pain-free knee *and* the pain stays consistent during the test.

Option 2: There is a difference in muscle strength between the knee with pain and the pain-free knee *and* in many cases the pain gets worse during the test.

In option 1, the test confirms that the pain is from the tear. Since muscles are not associated with the cause of pain, there is no reason to believe that there would be a decrease in strength of these muscles when tested. Also, the pain wouldn't increase because the tear is consistent no matter which muscle is working. Conversely, in option 2, we see that this *is* related to a muscle. Let's say that the cause of the knee pain is a hamstring strain in which the tendon that attaches the hamstrings to the knee is the tissue emitting the pain. If you were to muscle test the hamstrings, you should expect to find a major decrease in strength compared with the unaffected knee. You could also expect an increase in pain elicited by the testing of the hamstring.

So, very simply put, if pain is elicited and muscle weakness is identified when tested, this implies that the meniscal tear identified on the MRI is simply a degenerative tear that most likely has nothing to do with the knee pain.

Another reason for muscle testing is to figure out which muscles other than the one emitting the pain might be strained. By testing each muscle associated with the painful muscle, you can figure out all the muscles that need to be strengthened in order to regain proper function.

The final reason to perform muscle testing is to examine the strength of opposing muscles. This helps confirm when a muscle imbalance is the cause of a strained and painful muscle. To understand the importance of this, let's go back to our knee pain example. If you have pain around your kneecap and you have confirmed that the cause is muscular, not structural, you now have to determine which muscle is causing the pain. To do this, you will have to test all—or in this case, both—of the muscles that run by and affect the position of the kneecap: the quadriceps and the hamstrings. If one is stronger than the other, then you've found your muscle weakness. If the quads are stronger than the hamstrings, this allows the quads to shorten. Once shortened, they pull more intensely on their attachment to the kneecap. This causes the kneecap to be excessively compressed in the knee joint, creating irritation and pain. Conversely, if the hamstrings are stronger than the quads, you could postulate that because of the weakness of the quads, there is decreased upward force being created on the kneecap, allowing the kneecap to float slightly more up and to the side of the knee joint. Since the quads align more to the outside of the knee joint, the floating kneecap can now move more laterally in the knee joint, causing it to impact the lateral boundary of the knee joint, leading to irritation and pain.

This brings me to the next step in our testing process: checking out flexibility.

TECHNIQUE 3: FLEXIBILITY TEST

Because it is never smart to depend on only one test to provide a diagnosis, I use the flexibility test to confirm which muscle should be strengthened. It is also critical in understanding whether a strained muscle is at the proper length. If the muscle is overextended or shortened, the exercises that will help it are different.

Most therapists learned the length-tension ratio to get through school but never fully appreciate the significance of the law in their work. The length-tension ratio states that a muscle creates its greatest force at the middle length of the muscle. If a muscle is shortened too much or at an overstretched length, it loses its ability to create force. To remedy a muscle weakness, you have to exercise the muscle in a way that works to bring it back to the ideal length.

For example, if you're suffering from a hamstring strain, the natural response is to say that the correct treatment is to strengthen the hamstrings. But you first have to look at the length of the hamstring. If the hamstring strain is severe enough, you are going to find that the muscle has an increased tone enough to shorten the muscle to where it cannot be stretched to the normal range. If the hamstring is shortened, then strengthening the hamstring at this length will only cause it to shorten further. The shortened position will cause the muscle to lose the ability to create force, and the muscle will continue to be susceptible to straining with the mildest of force requirements based on the functional tasks of the patient. To fully resolve the pain brought about by the hamstring strain, you must first strengthen the quad muscle. This will create enough opposing force to stretch the hamstring muscle out to its optimal length. Only then can you strengthen the hamstring muscle.

I have treated a number of patients who had recurrent hamstring strains for years. They were treated by other therapists, and the treatment consisted mostly of hamstring-strengthening exercises. The hamstrings never developed full strength because they were always in a shortened position and therefore were always susceptible to strain.

Flexibility testing is a key to understanding the existing length of a muscle. Understanding where that length falls in the length-tension ratio is the key to knowing whether you initially want to strengthen the strained muscle or the opposing muscle.

TECHNIQUE 4: PALPATION

I truly believe that you cannot be a great diagnostician without having a thorough understanding of anatomy and an ability to pinpoint tissue with palpation. The work of palpation is simply in using your hands to examine the body—pressing on certain areas to see how pain is affected. And this can be hard if you aren't very familiar with anatomy. For example, when trying to determine which muscle is creating pain in the forearm, you need to be able to differentiate muscles that are very close to one another. In the gluteal region, you have muscles running superficial to deep. An ability to determine what level of tissue you are investigating and being able to follow the path of that muscle at different levels is a key to determining the tissue emitting the pain.

The ability to use palpation effectively can help you understand if the pain you are experiencing is point-tender (from the tissue you are pressing on) or referred (from a different location than where you are pressing)—and this in turn will help you identify the true cause of pain. For example, if someone is complaining of groin region pain, you can palpate the muscles associated with this area—the gracilis and the sartorius muscles—to establish if the pain is point-tender. If it is, the pain will increase when palpating one of these muscles. If the pain doesn't increase, the cause is not a strain of one of these muscles. A common diagnosis for groin region pain is referred pain from arthritis in the hip. This diagnosis can be tested by compressing the hip joint to cause further irritation. If this increases pain in the groin region, it confirms the diagnosis. Conversely, if no pain is experienced when compressing the hip joints, but it is experienced when pressing on the sartorius, gracilis, or hip flexor muscles, this reinforces that the cause of the pain is a strained muscle. It is that easy.

This simple test gives you one more confirmation of whether the pain is coming from a structural problem or a muscular weakness. In fact, palpation is a key test to refute a structural variation diagnosis—and to build confidence in an alternative diagnosis. Most patients understand point-tender versus referred pain, and when I have been forced to discredit an MRI result that promoted a structural cause, palpation was the key to making the patient believe me. This technique is easy to use and can provide lots of great information on the issue of point-tender versus referred pain.

TECHNIQUE 5: GAIT EVALUATION

Evaluating gait is an amazing technique that you can use to understand what's causing pain to occur anywhere from the back to the foot. If you can pinpoint something in someone's movement that isn't fluid or balanced, you can use this information to determine which muscles are causing the irregularity.

For example, if a patient has lower back pain on one side, I can watch them walk to see if they present with a hip drop on one side or the other. Finding a hip drop on the left side when the weight is on the right leg is a clear sign of a weak gluteus medius muscle (glute med). Since the gluteus medius muscle on one side works in conjunction with the lower back muscles on the other side to allow a person to stand on one leg during a walking cycle, an inability of the gluteus medius to perform its function correctly helps confirm its involvement in the cause of one-sided lower back pain.

I have found patients who circumducted a foot (moved it in a circular motion) as it was swung through from back to front while walking. This was a key finding that led me to see if they had a weakened anterior tibialis or hip flexor. The circumduction is caused by one of two things: (1) an inability of the patient to flex his or her foot enough to allow it to pass through during swing, or (2) a weak hip flexor that prevented the person from raising his or her knee high enough to allow the lower leg to swing through without the foot catching on the floor.

Clearly the gait evaluation doesn't give me the definitive answer about which muscle to focus on, but it does point me in the right direction. Remember, tests must be grouped; one single test cannot give you the final answer. So if I found a person who circumducted his or her foot while walking, I would then have to muscle test his or her anterior tibialis and hip flexors. I would also have to go back and see if there was a contributing factor, such as an injury, that would have led to a weakened anterior tibialis or hip flexor.

TECHNIQUE 6: POSTURAL ANALYSIS

Postural analysis is similar to gait evaluation in that it looks to identify possibly weak muscles by looking at how groups of muscles—and their various pulls on your body—are responsible for creating posture. There is a standard for normal posture that looks at how the bony landmarks—from the ear to the shoulder to the hip to the knee to the ankle—fall into alignment. If each of these stacks pretty clearly in a line when looking at someone from the side, this is considered good posture. To achieve this proper posture, the muscles in the front of the body must be generally equal in strength to the muscles in the back of the body.

Just as important as looking at posture from front to back is looking at posture from side to side. You want to see that the joints on one side of the body are equal in height to the joints on the other side of the body. To accomplish this, the muscles on both sides of the body must be equally strong.

If in either of these cases the muscles are not balanced, they will pull un-equally on their bony attachments. In the case of posture from front to back (a side view of you), this can lead to an altered posture known as forward shoulder posture in which the pec (chest), front shoulder, and biceps muscles are stronger than the muscles between the shoulder blades and the posterior shoulder and triceps muscles. This imbalance causes the shoulders to be drawn forward. With this imbalance the muscles in the back of the body become overstretched and lose their ability to create force, which can lead them to straining and emitting pain at the mid-back or neck—it can even create migraine headaches.

In the case of a postural abnormality when looking from side to side, you might find that one hip is higher than the other. This is a red flag that one of the hip muscles, called the gluteus medius muscle, has strained. This can cause the opposite-side lower back muscles to try to compensate, which can lead them to strain and shorten, pulling up the pelvis.

I have always found a postural evaluation to be a key to understanding what type of muscle weakness or imbalance may be present to create pain at any area of the body.

TECHNIQUE 7: BALANCE TESTING

The final technique that I regularly use is called balance testing. When some-one experiences pain on the lower half of only one side of the body, balance test-ing plays an important part in identifying the potential muscular cause.

When we walk, jog, climb stairs, or do any other type of locomotion, one foot remains on the floor while the other is lifted. The body's ability to support the leg being stood on, which is done through use of the gluteus medius, is key to normal function. If the glute med is weak, it often leads to muscle strains because your body compensates for this.

Balance testing confirms how well somebody is able to support himself or herself on one leg, thus indicating the strength of the glute med.

This test simply involves standing on one leg and then the other to see which one can be held for the longest period of time. People with a substantially weak-ened glute med may not be able to do this at all.

The other thing I look at during this test is what happens to someone's body when he or she does it. If the glute med is weak on one side because of a strain, the body will try to compensate by having the lower back muscles on the opposite side try to lift the pelvis up to keep it level. In most cases, when standing on the side with pain, the lower back muscles on the opposite side are not strong enough to achieve this goal and the pelvis on the opposite side starts to drop. If you notice the dropping pelvis—or if the person doing the test starts to fall to the side opposite the leg on which he or she is standing—this is a red flag for a strained glute med.

WHAT AFFECTS YOUR SYMPTOMS

While this isn't technically a clinical test, looking at what makes your symptoms better or worse is integral to understanding your pain. This evaluation can help you understand if your pain comes from a structural or muscular cause, which is why I delve into this topic with my patients.

The first question I often ask is: does your pain decrease temporarily if you have a massage but return in the not-too-distant future? If yes, this is a critical finding. If the cause of the pain were a structural variation, such as a herniated disc, stenosis, or nerve root impingement, all the massage in the world wouldn't help. Massage doesn't alter the structural variation and therefore would have no effect on your pain. The reduction in pain stems from the massage loosening and bringing blood to the muscles. The muscles heat up, and this allows them to lengthen.

Since the pain receptors sit in connective tissue that surrounds the muscle fibers, the lengthening of the muscles separates the pain receptors, decreasing the pain. Unfortunately, since nothing was done to resolve the imbalance in muscles that is the root cause of the symptoms, the symptoms return.

The same theory holds true if you find relief from things like a hot shower or some time in the sauna. The heat is allowing the muscles to loosen and bringing blood into them—nothing is being done that would fix a structural variation.

If you look at it from the other side—what makes the pain worse—you can see a similar pattern. If your pain is worse after resting or sleeping, consider that the muscle isn't being used. No warm blood is being pushed to it, and, therefore, the muscle shortens and contracts. This means that there is a concentration of the pain receptors that run along the muscle fibers that span the length of the muscle. As a result, there's more pain. I believe this is one of the more confusing symptoms associated with a muscular injury. Most people assume that it is when the muscle is being used that the pain should be experienced. Certainly in more serious cases where a strain or tear has occurred, pain will be experienced during use of the muscle. But as a general rule, pain occurs when the muscle has a chance to cool down and constrict to its shortest length. This concentrates the pain receptors found in the connective tissue that surrounds the muscle fibers, causing a higher degree of pain to be experienced.

So really take some time to think about your pain. What makes it better? What makes it worse? Just identifying these things can tell you quite a bit about the source of your pain.

READING YOUR SYMPTOMS

I know that much of what I've outlined above may sound intimidating because it's likely that you are not a trained medical professional. You don't know how to identify muscles and you aren't overly familiar with anatomy. But don't worry. In the second half of the book I will walk you step by step through how to do each and every bit of this in relation to the pain you are experiencing. This chapter is here as a reference so that when we move to the second half of the book and I begin to discuss these tests in defining different causes of pain, you have the ability to come back to reacquaint yourself with the tests and how they work.

These tests are necessary to create a complete narrative about what's causing your pain. This narrative allows you to explain which tissue is emitting the pain signal so it can be treated. Before I treat any patient, I create a narrative using exactly these techniques. And then I explain the issues in easy-to-understand terms. Just like I'll do in Part II of this book.

CHAPTER 4

UNDERSTANDING
COMMON
DIAGNOSES

Before we move on to figuring out whether muscle weaknesses or imbalances may be causing your pain, I'd like to go through some of the most common diagnoses that are given after diagnostic tests. If you've been to a medical professional to treat your pain, you've probably been told that one of the conditions listed in this chapter is the cause of your pain—but this may or may not be true.

I think it's important that you understand just what the diagnosis means, which is why I explain each one here. As I've stated, the vast majority of my patients are given invalid diagnoses based on diagnostic tests such as X-rays or MRIs. But when I looked at their symptoms it was obvious that the diagnosis could not be the cause of pain. The symptoms simply didn't match what would be expected if the structural problem was the cause of pain. In some cases the location of the pain was illogical because there was no connection between the structure and where the pain was. In other cases it was obvious that the pain was point-tender and not referred as would be required by the diagnosis. These mistakes were taking place in such a high percentage and were so clearly wrong that I realized nothing had been explained to the patient—they were simply given a diagnosis and expected to go along with it.

Sadly, I think there is a belief that most people are incapable of understanding what their symptoms mean when trying to determine the cause of their pain. I completely disagree. Once the majority of my patients described their symptoms and I correlated those with a proper diagnosis, they understood completely why their original diagnosis was incorrect.

Part of what I want to do in this book is give you the ability to determine what the cause of your pain is through interpreting your symptoms. In the existing medical model you are simply asked to accept the diagnosis in good faith, but I think it's better to explain what it means and what you should expect to find if it is correct. This truly puts the power back in your hands.

In this chapter, I provide a definition of the most common diagnoses associated with pain and then give you tests you can use to confirm or reject the diagnosis. Even if the simple test here confirms the diagnosis, I still recommend that you go through the chapters in Part II, doing the tests listed there, to double-check what you learned in this chapter.

The diagnoses are listed in alphabetical order along with the area of the body in which you're feeling pain. Feel free to skip around and only read the diagnosis (or diagnoses) that apply to you.

ADHESIVE CAPSULITIS (SHOULDER)

FROZEN SHOULDER

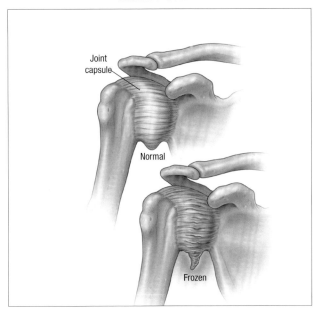

SHOULDER ANATOMY

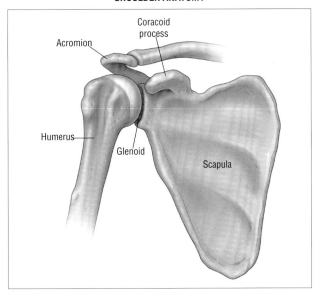

Adhesive capsulitis is one of the more common misdiagnoses of the shoulder. To understand the diagnosis, you have to understand the anatomy of the shoulder joint. The shoulder joint is composed of the upper arm bone and the end of the shoulder blade. Surrounding the joint is a joint capsule. The joint capsule provides a little stability to the joint, and it also allows for synovial fluid to be maintained in the joint. The synovial fluid acts as a lubricant to the joint while also providing nutrients to the cartilage on the ends of the bones.

When motion occurs at a joint, one of the bones that makes up the joint moves on the other bone to create the range of motion. The bones don't stay in a rigid position; they move in the joint. This is called gliding. In the shoulder joint, the amount of gliding that occurs is much greater because the range of motion that the joint goes through is so large. As a result of this large amount of gliding of the bones of the shoulder joint, the joint capsule is fairly lax.

If adhesive capsulitis develops, adhesions form on the joint capsule. This can result from systemic causes, such as infection, or as a result of trauma. The adhesions cause the joint capsule to lose its ability to stretch to allow for normal range of the shoulder joint. The bones of the shoulder joint can't glide normally because they are inhibited by the lack of flexibility of the joint capsule. With adhesive capsulitis there is a loss of range of motion of the shoulder joint not due to pain, although pain may be experienced, but from the inability of the arm bone to be raised in the shoulder joint due to the loss of flexibility of the joint capsule.

Testing an Adhesive Capsulitis Diagnosis: In a case of adhesive capsulitis, not only would you experience pain at the shoulder joint but you would also find a substantial decrease in range of motion—both active and passive motion. Understanding if your pain truly comes from adhesive capsulitis rather than a muscular cause comes through testing active and passive range of motion. If the cause of your shoulder pain is muscular based, you can find a decreased range of motion when you try to raise your arm (active) but not when someone else does it for you (passive). For adhesive capsulitis to be considered the cause of pain, there must also be an exactly equal loss of range of motion in both the active and passive test. When the person passively tries to raise the shoulder and is stopped, it must also feel as if there is resistance at the end point, indicating that something is structurally preventing the shoulder from moving any farther.

ARTHRITIS/OSTEOARTHRITIS/BONE-ON-BONE (KNEE, SHOULDER, HIP)

ARTHRITIC KNEE

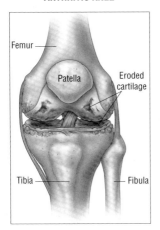

ARTHRITIC HIP

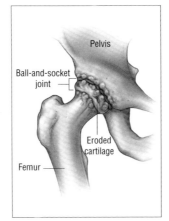

ARTHRITIC SHOULDER

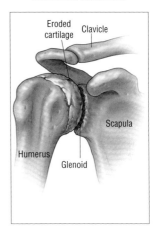

Generally when doctors use an X-ray to diagnose arthritis, they are talking about osteoarthritis, a mechanical issue, and not one of the other forms of arthritis that are inflammatory, such as rheumatoid or psoriatic arthritis. Osteoarthritis is by far the most common form of arthritis. This is why I'm using the terms interchangeably in this section.

Arthritis/osteoarthritis is one of the most common diagnoses given in response to knee, shoulder, and hip pain. Osteoarthritis is typically a result of the surfaces of a joint wearing down. It is a progressive mechanical—again, not inflammatory—condition, and its slow progression means that the variations in joint structures occur over such a long period of time that pain is not generally a side effect. Certainly as you get older there is a greater chance that you will have some form of osteoarthritis, but studies have shown that there are almost as many people with arthritis who have no pain as those with pain.

To fully understand the diagnosis of arthritis, you have to go back to the definition of a joint. A joint is nothing more than a pivot point where motion occurs. The surfaces that make up joints are designed to align in a particular way in order to disperse the pressures associated with movement. This alignment is kept intact by the muscles that pass by the joints. If the muscles are strong and balanced, the joint works as it is supposed to. What I mean by *balanced* is that for every muscle there is an opposing muscle. For example, you have the front upper arm muscle (the biceps), which is opposed by the posterior upper arm muscle (the triceps).

When these muscles are balanced in strength, the alignment of the joint they support stays true. When that joint is called on to move or assist in performing a functional task, that force is dispersed evenly across the entire joint. When the joint surfaces do not align properly, force is not evenly supported. So if there were a misalignment of the bones that make up the knee and only 80 percent of the bone surface was aligned, you would have 80 percent of the joint supporting 100 percent of the body weight that passes through it. Over time that 80 percent of the joint would not be able to sustain the pressure and the surfaces—more specifically, the cartilage at the end of the bone—would begin to wear down. When the cartilage wears down, bone can be exposed. The body will either wear away the bone or grow excessive bone. This is arthritis.

I like to give the analogy of the rust on a bridge to help people better understand what the diagnosis of arthritis means. Most bridges have large deposits of rust on the structural steel of which they are constructed. Yet most of us will confidently go over the bridge without fear because we assume that, although there is a structural variation to the steel, the integrity of the steel and the bridge is still intact. The same goes with arthritis and joints. As long as the integrity of the joint is still intact, the finding of arthritis is insignificant.

How do you know if the integrity of the joint is intact? If it moves through full range of motion. So to know if arthritis is the cause of your pain, you have to look at range of motion. If an arthritic change has occurred, but the joint is still able to function, then arthritis should be discounted as a cause.

I have noted this before, but I want to say it again here: because osteoarthritis is not an inflammatory response, the use of anti-inflammatory medicines will not resolve your pain. Whether it is NSAIDs (nonsteroidal anti-inflammatory drugs) or steroidal medications, they are given under the premise that the cause of your pain is an inflammatory response. A common procedure performed by physicians in the treatment of arthritis is the use of cortisone shots—and this treatment works for a short time, but only because it is treating the symptom of pain, not the cause. Cortisone shots, steroidal anti-inflammatory medications, are typically paired with lidocaine, which provides pain relief by dulling the nervous system's ability to sense pain. The anesthetic is what provides the pain relief, not the lessening of inflammation. These shots and medications create the false perception that inflammation is the true cause of pain, which leads to long-term treatment of symptoms rather than a resolution of the problem.

Testing an Arthritis Diagnosis at the Knee: The only time osteoarthritis can create knee pain is when the joint's range of motion is compromised, so this is what must be tested. For those people who have gotten an X-ray and a bone-on-bone diagnosis, this is especially important because a total knee replacement is often suggested as the treatment. In this scenario, there is no question that there is decreased joint space and that some form of deterioration has occurred. But the question about whether this is the cause of your pain is whether there is absolutely no joint space, as the phrase *bone-on-bone* represents. If there is no space, there will be a loss in both active and passive range of motion.

Just about every movable joint has a space that separates the ends of the bones that make up the joint. The joint space is usually maintained by cartilage or a meniscus. The purpose of the joint space is to give the bones the ability to glide on one another. The bones that make up a joint actually shift in the joint to allow the joint to move. If there were no joint space and the bones were touching, there would be no ability for the bones to glide, which would mean that no motion could take place in the joint.

To test your active range of motion, first move your unaffected knee through its range of motion. See how much you can straighten and bend it. Then try the painful knee. If there is a substantial loss of range of motion in your ability to straighten or bend your painful knee, this shows a loss of active range of motion. Then test your passive range of motion: have someone else try to straighten and bend your painful knee. If the same substantial loss of range of motion is evident passively and if it feels as though a bone touching a bone is the limiting factor, this is confirmation that bone on bone exists and that this is the cause of the knee pain. However, if the active range of motion is limited because of pain and the passive range of motion is full or almost full, this indicates that it is not.

Another thing to examine is where the pain at the knee joint is being experienced. There are two joints that make up the knee: the joint between the kneecap and the thigh bone and the joint between the thigh bone and the lower leg bone. If bone on bone is the cause of your knee pain, the pain must be experienced at the joint between the thigh bone and the lower leg bone. This can be felt by identifying the joint line (there is a medial and lateral joint line) and pressing on the line to see if pain is elicited. If the pain is around your kneecap, not at the joint line, this signals that bone on bone is not the cause of the pain.

SURFACE KNEE JOINT LINE

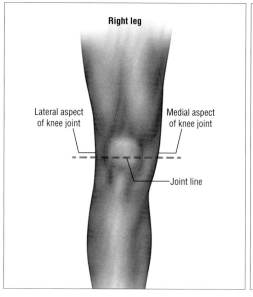

ANATOMY OF THE KNEE

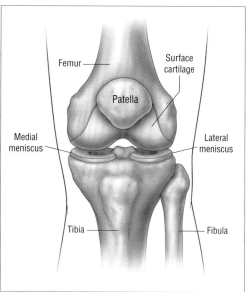

To confirm if a simple diagnosis of osteoarthritis or the more severe diagnosis of bone on bone is correct, look at range of motion (both active and passive) and perform palpation to determine exactly where the pain is being experienced.

Testing an Arthritis Diagnosis at the Shoulder: The easiest way to confirm or dispute a diagnosis of arthritis/osteoarthritis at the shoulder is to see if you have full range of motion—both active and passive.

The typical diagnosis of arthritis at the shoulder joint pertains to one specific bony landmark: the acromion process.

ANATOMY OF SHOULDER

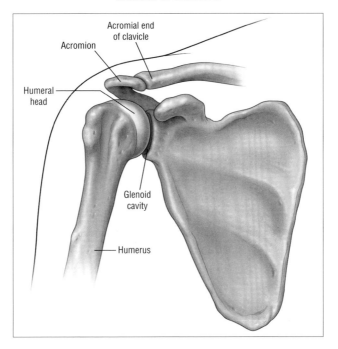

The acromion creates the top border of the shoulder joint, and the arm bone sits below this bony protuberance. Pain at the shoulder typically results in an X-ray of the joint, and this X-ray often shows one of two things: (1) an arthritic change in the form of a bone spur that extends down from the acromion into the shoulder joint or (2) a hooked shape to the acromion process. In both cases the cause of pain is determined to be the altered bony landmark entering the space between the acromion process and the head of the humerus (upper arm bone). The key to understanding the mechanics of shoulder movement is that when the arm bone is raised, the space between the head of the arm bone and the acromion process must be maintained. This space, called the subacromial space, allows the upper arm bone to move freely in the shoulder joint without creating pain.

As I mentioned above, testing this diagnosis depends on evaluating active and passive range of motion when raising the arm in front of you. To test your active range of motion, first raise your unaffected arm up in front of you and then up to the side, moving the shoulder through its range of motion. See how high you can raise it. Then try the arm with the painful shoulder. If there is a substantial loss of range of motion on the painful side, this shows a loss of active range of motion. Then test your passive range of motion: have someone else try to raise the arm on the side with your painful shoulder. If the same substantial loss of range of motion is evident passively and if it feels like a bone touching a bone is the limiting factor, this is confirmation that arthritis could be the cause of your pain. However, if the active range of motion is limited because of pain and the passive range of motion is full or almost full, this indicates that it is not.

The diagnosis of bone on bone for the shoulder is one of the most surprising ones I hear for pain in this region. In the hip or knee joint, bone on bone is a little more probable because of the weight being put on the joint every day—as a person stands, walks, runs, hikes, climbs stairs, and so on. The gravitational (compressive) force placed on these joints can lead to a breakdown of the joint surfaces unless the proper strength and muscle balance is maintained. But this is not a factor at the shoulder joint. In fact, the shoulder joint has to deal with just the opposite forces (distractive): the weight of the arm bone and musculature is trying to pull down on the shoulder joint separating the joint surfaces, rather than compressing them. While I cannot deny that X-ray sometimes shows a decreased joint space between the upper bone and shoulder bone, only the testing of range of motion can truly determine if in fact the joint has become bone-on-bone.

Testing an Arthritis Diagnosis at the Hip: The easiest way to determine if the cause of the pain is coming from arthritis of the hip joint is to perform a compression test of the joint. You'll need someone to help you do this. Lie on your side, with the painful hip up. Have your helper find the hip joint, place his or her palms one on top of the other, and then press down on the head of the femur (the bone that sticks out when you're feeling for the hip joint). This compresses the joint surfaces in the hip joint. If the pain were coming from an arthritic change in the joint, pain would be experienced. And if bone on bone were the cause of your pain, this test would cause very severe pain.

PELVIS AND HIP

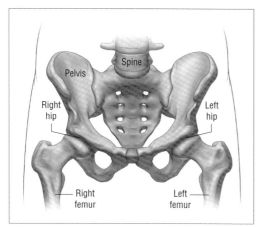

HIP COMPRESSION TEST

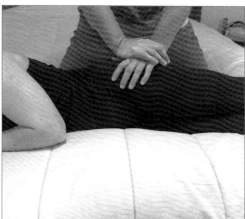

The other confirmatory test is to check both active and passive ranges of motion of the hip joint. To do this, lie on your back on a flat surface and pull the knee on your painful side toward your chest as far as you can. Then have somebody else move your leg for you. This test looks at the range of motion of the knee into hip flexion.

Then you will test the hip's range of motion in abduction. To do this, move the leg associated with your painful hip region out to the side as far as you can go. Then do the test again with somebody else moving your leg.

In both the test for hip flexion and the test for abduction, the movements you make on your own test the active range of motion. Those done by your helper test the passive range of motion.

If there is a loss of both the active and passive ranges of motion, the loss is roughly at the same location in the range, and the limiting feeling is that a bone is touching another bone and inhibiting any further motion, this is another indicator that arthritis is the cause of the hip region pain.

In the case of the hip being bone-on-bone, there would have to be a substantial loss of range of motion both actively and passively. In my experience, very few people experience this loss of range of motion.

BULGING DISC (NECK, MID-BACK, LOWER BACK)

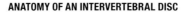

ANATOMY OF AN INTERVERTEBRAL DISC

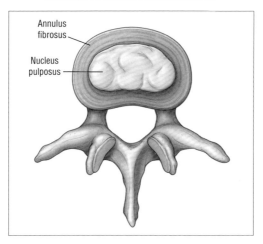

Annulus
fibrosus

Nucleus
pulposus

A bulging disc is the least severe variation you'll find of problems in the vertebral discs of the spine—a herniated or ruptured disc is much more severe. To understand what a bulging disc is, you'll need to understand the structure of the spine. The spine is composed of a spinal cord protected by 29 vertebrae; all but the sacral vertebrae are separated by a disc that has a gel-like substance called the nucleus pulposus in its center. The gel is surrounded by a connective tissue covering called the annulus. The gel is designed to take the force of gravity pushing down on you and your spine. And the annulus is designed to keep the gel in place in the center of the disc. When a person has bad posture due to muscle weakness or imbalances, the forces on the spine can be altered and the force of gravity pressing down on the individual and his or her spine may not be centered. This can cause excessive forces to develop on one side of the spine or the other. These excessive forces—and in a few cases, structural disc malformations—lead the gel-like substance in the vertebral discs to shift off to one side of the spinal column. As long as the border of the gel is still inside the spinal column—even though it is no longer centered—it is considered a bulging disc.

The thing to understand about these types of abnormalities is that they are very common. The variation from being centered in the spinal column to off to one side occurs over a long period. Since there is no impact on any other tissue, typically no symptoms are expected.

Testing the Diagnosis of a Bulging Disc at the Neck, Mid-Back, or Lower Back:
The finding of a bulging disc is considered to be very benign and not the cause of pain as a general rule. Thus no test is required.

BURSITIS (SHOULDER, HIP)

SHOULDER BURSA

HIP BURSA

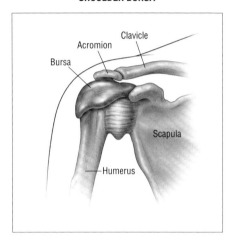
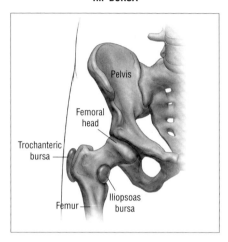

This is a very common diagnosis for people who have shoulder or hip pain. A broader understanding of anatomy will help you decide if bursitis could be the cause of your pain.

To fully understand, first you need to know that bursa is a pouch of fluid designed to limit friction and irritation between tissues that might touch each other when movement is occurring. For instance, if the tendon of a muscle passes close to a bone, a bursa would be between them to prevent irritation of either tissue.

In the shoulder joint, the main bursa is found below the acromion process. It is called the subacromial bursa. The bursa sits in this area because several tendons, including the biceps and rotator cuff tendons, pass between the upper arm bone and the acromion process. The bursa prevents irritation of these tendons while shoulder motion is occurring. If the bursa were to become inflamed because of improper shoulder function, the bursa would swell.

This is also true for the hip; an obvious pouch of fluid would be present surrounding the hip joint.

In my 20 years of treating patients, I have seen maybe one or two instances where bursitis is the cause of pain in either the hip or the shoulder.

Testing the Diagnosis of a Bursitis at the Shoulder: To test the diagnosis of bursitis at the shoulder, you will look and feel for swelling at the shoulder. In the shoulder, there should be a pouch of fluid protruding out from either side of the acromion process.

Since the bursa of the shoulder sits within the shoulder joint, the range of motion of the shoulder will also be inhibited, so you must evaluate active and passive ranges of motion when raising the arm. To test your active range of motion, first raise your unaffected arm up in front of you and then up to the side, moving the shoulder through its range of motion. See how high you can raise it. Then try the arm with your painful shoulder. If there is a substantial loss of range of motion on the painful side, this shows a loss of active range of motion. Then test your passive range of motion: have someone else try to raise the arm on the side with your painful shoulder. If the same substantial loss of range of motion is evident passively, this is confirmation that bursitis could be the cause of your pain. However, if the active range of motion is decreased by pain but the passive range of motion is equal to or almost equal to the unaffected side, this indicates that it is not.

Testing the Diagnosis of a Bursitis at the Hip: To test the diagnosis of bursitis at the hip, you will look and feel for swelling around the hip joint.

Since the bursa of the hip sits within the hip joint, the range of motion of the hip will also be inhibited, so you must evaluate active and passive ranges of motion for the hip joint. To do this, lie on your back on a flat surface and pull the knee on your painful side toward your chest as far as you can. Then have somebody else move your leg for you. This test looks at the range of motion of the knee into hip flexion.

Then you will test the hip's range of motion in abduction. To do this, move the leg associated with your painful hip region out to the side as far as you can go. Then do the test again with somebody else moving your leg.

In both the test for hip flexion and the test for abduction, the movements you make on your own test the active range of motion. Those done by your helper test the passive range of motion.

If there is a loss of both the active and passive ranges of motion, the loss is roughly at the same location in the range, and the limiting feeling is that something is inhibiting any further motion, this is another indicator that bursitis could be the cause of the hip region pain. However, if the active range of motion is decreased by pain, but the passive range of motion is equal to or almost equal to the unaffected side, this indicates that it is not.

COMPRESSION FRACTURE (NECK, MID-BACK, LOWER BACK)

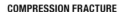

COMPRESSION FRACTURE

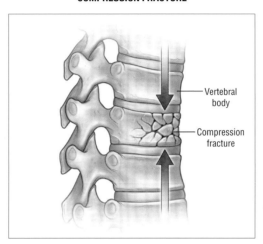

Vertebral body

Compression fracture

A compression fracture is a structural variation to a vertebra in the spinal column that typically occurs over time. In essence, the bone of the vertebra cracks as a result of long-term pressure. This diagnosis, which is obtained through the use of an X-ray, is sometimes given in relation to neck, mid-back, or lower back pain, and it is commonly given to elderly people as a reason for their pain.

Compression fractures are another one of those structural abnormalities that often don't emit pain signals because their progression is so slow. However, there are incidences when a fall can lead to an acute compression fracture causing pain.

In either case, the important thing to understand is that the pain being experienced would be isolated to the vertebra that was fractured—the area of pain would be very small. In general, a compression fracture cannot account for more widespread pain in the neck or the back. And in the case of the fall-induced compression fracture, you wouldn't have experienced the pain before the fall.

Testing the Diagnosis of a Compression Fracture at the Neck, Mid-Back, or Lower Back: If you have been diagnosed with a compression fracture, no matter which part of your neck or back, the first thing you need to do is have someone palpate, or feel, where you are experiencing pain. If the area is vast in size or simply in a location away from the vertebrae where the compression fracture was found, the fracture cannot be the cause of your pain. The pain caused by a compression fracture must be strictly limited to the vertebra that has been fractured.

FRACTURE (KNEE, SHOULDER, HIP)

There are some instances where a fracture is identified as the cause of knee or shoulder pain. If a trauma occurred, certainly there is a good chance that this is the real cause. However, if some time has passed since the injury and you're still experiencing pain, it is likely coming from a muscle strain or imbalance that resulted from the injury.

If a fracture is indeed the cause of the pain, there are two things you must understand. (1) In most cases there must be a trauma associated with the pain. There are those exceptions where metabolic dysfunction can account for a fracture with the most minimal of forces. But most likely, if you cannot recall a specific incident or time frame when the pain began, it is likely not a fracture causing your pain. (2) The pain would be located specifically where the facture is. Just as in the compression fracture, the area of pain would be relatively small.

Testing the Diagnosis of a Fracture at the Knee: If you did experience trauma, I can't stress this enough: go get an X-ray. If trauma was experienced and pain developed immediately or shortly thereafter, an X-ray could not only help determine the cause of the pain but also lead to the proper treatment.

ANATOMY OF THE KNEE

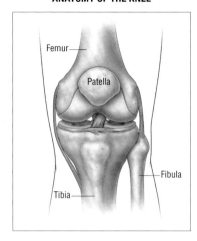

ANTERIOR AND POSTERIOR MUSCULATURE OF THE KNEE

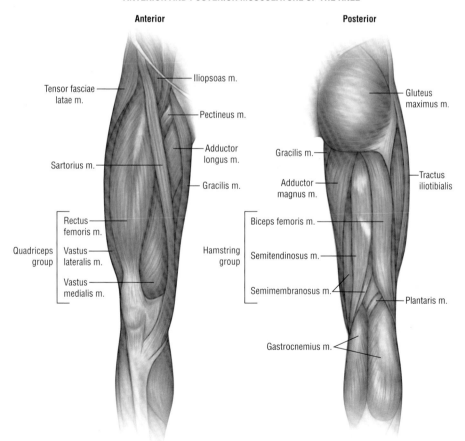

However, if no trauma was experienced and pain develops, the best way to identify the cause of the pain is palpation. The knee joint is composed of two joints: the joint between the kneecap and the thigh bone and the joint between the thigh bone and the lower leg bone. There are a variety of muscles that attach and pass the knee joint. The ability to identify each of these tissues is key to determining which one is emitting the pain signal you are experiencing.

If you are told that you have a tibial plateau fracture, then you should feel pain at the joint line between the thigh bone and lower leg bone. If you are told that your pain is coming from a fractured patella (kneecap), then you can expect to feel pain when you palpate the kneecap.

In order to confirm the fracture as the cause of the pain, you will also want to palpate the muscles surrounding the fracture to verify that they are not emitting pain. If a patella fracture is the cause of your knee region pain, then palpating the quadriceps muscle or quad tendon should not emit pain. If a tibial plateau fracture is the cause of your pain, then feeling the joint line between the thigh bone and lower leg bone should emit pain, but feeling the attachment of the hamstring tendon or other muscle attachments near the joint line should not emit pain.

Testing the Diagnosis of a Fracture at the Shoulder: If you did experience trauma, I can't stress this enough: go get an X-ray. If trauma was experienced and pain developed immediately or shortly thereafter, an X-ray could not only help determine the cause of the pain but also lead to the proper treatment.

ANATOMY OF THE SHOULDER JOINT

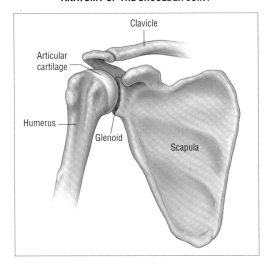

MUSCULATURE OF THE NECK AND UPPER BACK

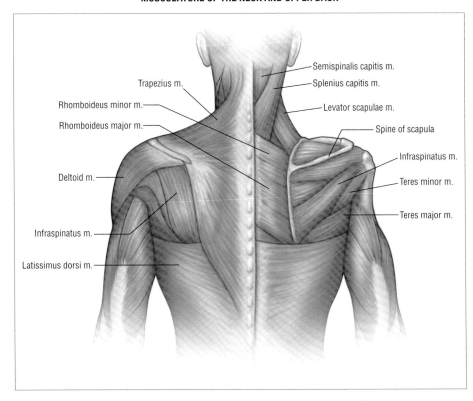

The concern that a fracture is causing your pain is also heightened if you had full range of motion of the shoulder before the trauma and after there is a substantial loss of range of motion. If no trauma was experienced and pain develops at the shoulder region, then palpation is a good way to begin to identify which tissue is emitting the pain signal: whether it is a fractured bone, a strained muscle, or even an inflamed bursa.

Palpate the tissues in your shoulder region. It is important to be able to differentiate all the tissues in the shoulder region, including the bony structures and muscles. If your pain increases while pressing on these non-bone tissues, there is a good chance that the pain is not coming from a fracture. If you feel the humerus, or upper arm bone, and you can locate a point on the bone where pain is being emitted and this spot is fairly small, this could indicate that the pain is from a fracture. The same is true with the acromion process. If you have not yet had an X-ray, and you think you might have a fracture, please go get an X-ray.

Testing the Diagnosis of a Fracture at the Hip: If you experienced a trauma and now have hip pain plus you have an inability to bear weight, I highly recommend getting an X-ray to determine whether a fracture has occurred.

ANATOMY OF THE HIP AND PELVIS

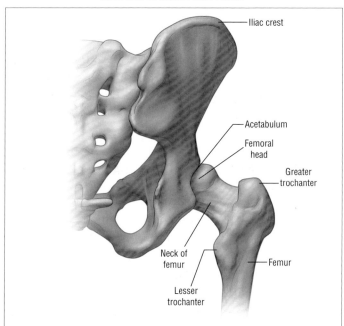

If no trauma has occurred and you are experiencing hip pain, the best way to confirm that the cause of pain is a fracture is through palpating, or feeling, the tissues in the hip region. If your pain increases while pressing on these tissues, there is a good chance that the pain is not coming from a fracture. If you press on the femur (thigh bone) near the hip region, and you can locate a point on the bone where pain is being emitted and this spot is fairly small, this could indicate that the pain is from a fracture.

HIP COMPRESSION TEST

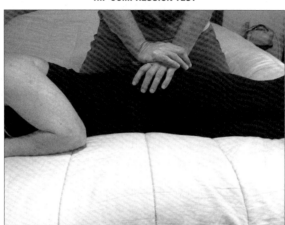

If you have somebody perform a compression test to the hip joint in which he or she applies pressure and you get pain in the joint, this is another indicator that the cause of the pain in the hip region could be a fracture. If you have not yet had an X-ray, and you think you might have a fracture, please go get an X-ray.

HERNIATED DISC (NECK, MID-BACK, LOWER BACK)

A herniated disc is a more severe variation you might find in problems associated with the vertebral discs of the spine. To understand what a herniated disc is, you'll need to understand the structure of the spine. The spine is composed of the spinal cord protected by 29 vertebrae; all but the sacral vertebrae are separated by a disc that has a gel-like substance called the nucleus pulposus in its center. The gel is surrounded by a connective tissue covering called the annulus. The gel is designed to take the force of gravity pushing down on you and your spine. And the annulus is designed to keep the gel in place in the center of the disc. When a person has bad posture due to muscle weakness or imbalances, the forces on the spine can be altered and the force of gravity pressing down on the individual and his or her spine may not be centered. This can cause excessive forces to develop on one side of the spine or the other. These excessive forces—and, in a few cases, structural disc malformations—shift the gel-like substance in the vertebral discs. Most often the gel is shifted to the front or the back of the vertebral column and off to one side. If the shift is great enough that the gel-like substance is no longer confined to within the spinal column, you have a herniated disc. The gel-like substance is now protruding out of the spinal column, but it is still fully encased in the annulus.

It is possible for a herniated disc to cause pain because the shifted gel may come into contact with other tissues. The tissue with the greatest potential to be impacted by a herniated disc is a nerve root, an extension of the spinal cord in the spinal column. These nerve roots then extend out from the spinal cord and column through little tunnels called foramens and impact sensation in the arms, legs, and torso.

What is important to understand is that the disc is made of fibro cartilage, which is a tough, dense form of cartilage designed to absorb a lot of force. This type of tissue does not have pain receptors in it; therefore, the disc itself cannot cause pain. The only question is whether the herniated disc is impinging on another tissue. Studies have shown that roughly 70 percent of the population has a bulging or herniated disc with no pain, so merely having a herniated disc should not be thought of as the cause of pain. You must look at the bigger picture.

Testing the Diagnosis of a Herniated Disc at the Neck, Mid-Back, or Lower Back: The key to knowing if a herniated disc is causing your pain is understanding just how the nerves work. The nerve roots innervate specific areas of skin called dermatomes to provide sensation. If an impinged nerve root from a herniated disc is the cause of the symptom being experienced, the symptom must be in the area of skin innervated by the nerve root. It must be within the area and nowhere else. So you must assess if the pain you are experiencing is in the proper place based on which disc is herniated. You can do this by using the chart opposite to see where on the body the nerves associated with your herniation innervate. If the pain is outside that area, the diagnosis that a herniated disc is the cause of your pain is likely incorrect.

DERMATOMAL CHART OF THE BODY

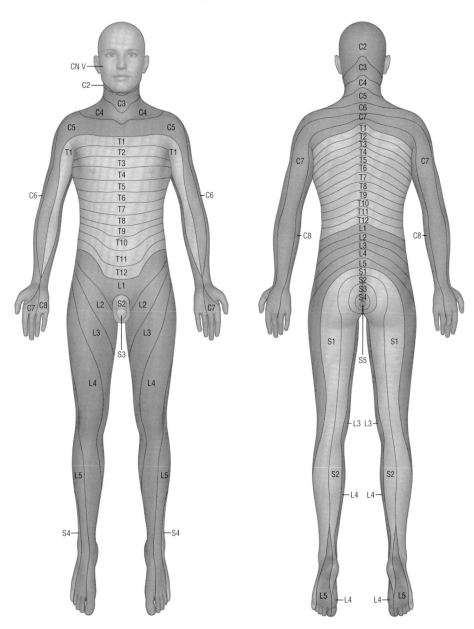

The other thing to look for in testing whether a herniated disc is the cause of pain is whether the pain or symptom being experienced is referred or point-tender. Does the pain you are experiencing get worse if you push on the herniated vertebra, or does it get worse if you press where the pain is experienced? If the pain gets worse by pressing directly on it, but not when you press on the vertebra, this is an indication that the herniated disc is not the cause of your pain.

IMPINGEMENT SYNDROME (SHOULDER)

ANATOMY OF THE SHOULDER JOINT

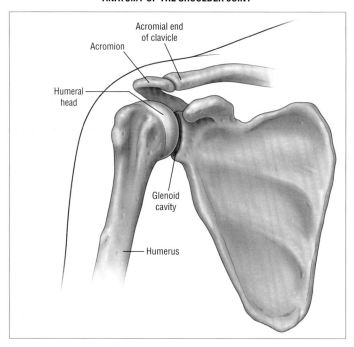

Impingement syndrome is a general diagnosis, which means that it can be caused by a variety of things. Impingement syndrome can occur from both structural and muscular causes. *Impingement syndrome* is basically a term that states that the space between the acromion process and the head of the upper arm bone (humerus) in the shoulder joint is being impeded on. The key to understanding the mechanics of shoulder movement is that when the arm bone is raised, the space between the head of the arm bone and the acromion process must be maintained. This space, called the subacromial space, allows the upper arm bone to move freely in the shoulder joint without creating pain.

Many doctors state that the cause of impingement syndrome is due to one of three things: (1) arthritis, (2) an altered shape in the acromion process that points down into the subacromial space, or (3) an inflamed bursa, which is causing a loss of space. With any of these diagnoses, the doctor is simply saying that there is a loss of subacromial space.

As with all structural causes of pain, a loss in both active and passive ranges of motion would be expected. If the structure is still functionally intact, meaning the shoulder can still move through full range of motion, the structural causes of impingement syndrome are likely not the cause of your pain.

Testing an Impingement Syndrome Diagnosis at the Shoulder: Testing this diagnosis lies in evaluating active and passive range of motion when raising the arm. To test your active range of motion, first raise your unaffected arm up in front of you and then up to the side, moving the shoulder through its range of motion. See how high you can raise it. Then try the arm with the painful shoulder. If there is a substantial loss of range of motion on the painful side, this shows a loss of active range of motion. Then test your passive range of motion: have someone else try to raise the arm on the side with the painful shoulder. If the same substantial loss of range of motion is evident passively, this is confirmation that a structural change could be the cause of your pain. However, if the active range of motion is limited by pain but the passive range of motion is the same or almost the same as the unaffected side, then the possibility of a structural cause of impingement such as arthritis or bursitis is unlikely.

LABRAL TEAR (HIP, SHOULDER)

HIP JOINT LABRAL TEAR

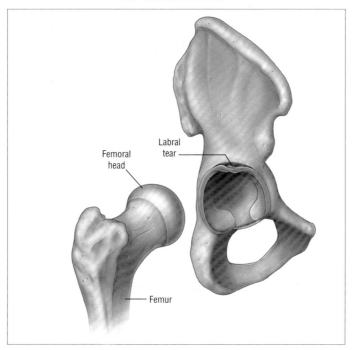

SHOULDER LABRAL TEAR

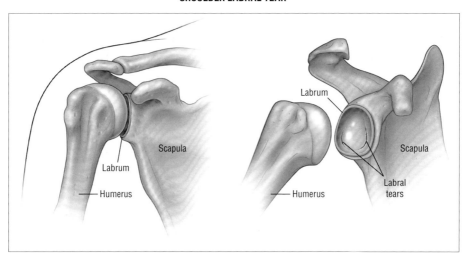

A torn labrum is sometimes diagnosed as the cause of hip or shoulder pain. This is usually established by a positive finding on an MRI. However, it is possible that this tear is not the cause of your pain, because a labral tear can be degenerative, occurring over such a long period of time that it doesn't produce symptoms.

The labrum is a piece of cartilage made of fibrocartilage, a tough, dense form of cartilage designed to absorb a lot of force. This type of tissue does not have pain receptors in it. This cartilage not only absorbs pressure, it also stabilizes the joint and deepens it, allowing for the bones to glide properly against one another.

In the hip, the labrum is an extension of the socket of the hip joint. In the shoulder, it surrounds the end of the shoulder blade that makes up one-half of the shoulder joint, called the glenoid fossa.

If the labrum is torn, the cartilage that allows the joint to move smoothly could be caught between the head of the humerus (upper arm bone) and the shoulder blade at the shoulder joint or between the thigh bone and pelvis at the hip joint. It is for this reason that the most common indicator of a labral tear is if the joint has a tendency to catch or lock. A common description of this at the shoulder joint is that you put your arm up on something and when you try to move it, you find that it is stuck; you are unable to lower your arm and your shoulder hurts. The same type of symptom can be experienced at the hip. With a labral tear, you would expect the hip joint to lock intermittently, causing an inability to move the joint along with increased hip pain.

In either of these situations, movement can generally be restored by manually manipulating the shoulder or hip joint to cause it to release.

If this type of symptom is not experienced, the tear is likely degenerative. It would not cause symptoms because the extended period of time over which it has occurred included scarring that prevents the loose piece of cartilage from moving; thus, it can't get stuck in the joint.

In either of these regions, it is also important to recognize that the labral tears that create symptoms are the result of a traumatic incident, like an awkward fall or some type of impact to the joint. If you can't recall a traumatic event or time frame for when the pain started, the cause of your pain is likely not a labral tear.

Testing a Labral Tear Diagnosis at the Hip or the Shoulder: The primary test that can be done is to move the hip or shoulder joint through its range of motion. Move the shoulder in front of you and to the side of you, raising and lowering your arm. Then move your arm in circles at the shoulder. At the hip, try to bend the hip in front of you and to the side of you. Try to rotate the hip inward and outward. Through these varied movements, if a labral tear is the cause of pain, you should be able to create a situation in which your joint locks. If no locking or catching can be elicited, this is an indicator that a labral tear is not the cause of your pain.

LIGAMENT TEAR (KNEE)

I'm not going to go in depth discussing ligament tears, such as the ACL (anterior cruciate ligament) and PCL (posterior cruciate ligament), because these should not be the diagnosis for any joint pain that is not associated with a specific traumatic event. If your pain is not associated with an excessive force that moved your joint *past* its normal range of motion, you should discard this diagnosis immediately.

The reason I do want to talk about it here is because there is a way to avoid surgery if you have torn a ligament in your knee. Unfortunately, there is little that can be done to heal a torn ligament, as ligaments are avascular—meaning that they have no blood supply—so once injured, they can't grow new tissue. This is why so many people opt for surgery, which involves a surgeon manually grafting new tissue from another part of your body, such as a tendon, or using cadaver tissue to replace the ligament.

The reason you don't necessarily need surgery is because ligaments are only designed to come into play at the end of a joint's range of motion. When a joint is going through normal range of motion, the ligaments that surround the joint are lax. It is only at the end range of motion when the ligament becomes taut to prevent the joint from going farther. While this is good backup to have, strong muscles surrounding the joint make it less necessary to keep the joint from moving beyond its natural range of motion. Each joint is supported by associated muscle groups, so as long as these muscles are strong, they provide the stability you will need. For instance, when you are standing or walking, the muscles on the sides of the ankle provide stability; the ligaments are lax unless you twist your ankle excessively. The stronger the muscles, the less likely the need for the ligament to come into play. So before opting for surgery, I recommend that you first exhaust every opportunity to strengthen the appropriate muscles that provide stability to your knee.

Testing a Ligament Tear Diagnosis at the Knee: As I noted, this should never be a diagnosis associated with a pain that has come on slowly—a trauma will need to have occurred. If a trauma has occurred and you are experiencing pain, and if a ligament is involved in creating the pain, some form of instability of the joint should be present. If pain and instability are present after a trauma, then I would certainly endorse the use of an MRI to identify which tissues have been damaged and are emitting the pain signal.

MENISCAL TEAR (KNEE)

MENISCAL TEAR IN THE KNEE

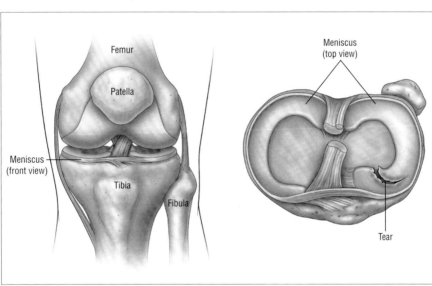

A meniscal tear is one of the most common positive diagnostic test findings established at the knee. There are a couple of things you need to understand about the structure of the knee in order to understand whether or not a meniscal tear could be the cause of your pain.

The first is that the meniscus is a structure found in the knee joint that works to support and protect the bottom of the thigh bone and the top of the lower leg bone. The meniscus is made of fibrocartilage that is designed to absorb the shock of weight bearing, and it is designed to take a lot of pressure; simply putting weight on the knee is not enough to cause the meniscus to tear. When the joint does not function properly, tearing is possible.

If you look at the way the thigh bone meets the lower leg bone, the knee works most efficiently when these two bones are in maximum alignment. When the thigh bone sits directly over the lower leg bone, weight is borne in a balanced way, spread over the maximum surface area possible. If there is a muscle imbalance or weakness, this can affect the positioning of the joint surfaces, changing the pressure applied to the surface areas of the meniscus. This excessive force can cause a deterioration of the meniscus, which can slowly cause a progressive tearing of the meniscus; however, this slow progress will not create pain. Only an acute meniscal tear due to trauma could cause a tear of the meniscal and adjacent tissues to create pain. Studies have shown that a large percentage of the population with no pain at the knee have meniscal tears present.

Another point to understand about the meniscus is that because of its shape, there are only certain types of movements that can create acute meniscal tears. Let's examine the appearance of the meniscus. Notice how the majority of the meniscus is flat except for the outer edge that runs from the front around the side to the back of the knee joint. The reason for this raised edge is that the knee joint is somewhat shallow. To increase the depth of the joint, the meniscus has this raised outer edge. It provides more depth to the joint, creating more stability when the joint is in motion. This raised portion, however, makes the meniscus more susceptible to being caught and torn. An acute meniscal tear that creates pain typically happens when the knee is forced into a position that affects this outer rim, which leads to portions of the meniscus being pulled away from its attachment to the tibia.

The most common causes of an acute meniscal tear are hyperextension of the knee (excessively straightening the knee), hyperflexing the knee (extreme bending of the knee), or weight bearing on the leg while twisting the knee with excessive force. These types of forces are usually associated with traumatic events. It is rare that common movements could cause the extent of force necessary to tear the meniscus. If you cannot remember a traumatic event that involved one of these movements, it is likely that the pain you are experiencing is not from a meniscal tear.

The pain caused by a meniscal tear should be experienced at the joint line—the space between the thigh bone and the lower leg bone.

SURFACE INDICATION OF THE KNEE JOINT LINE

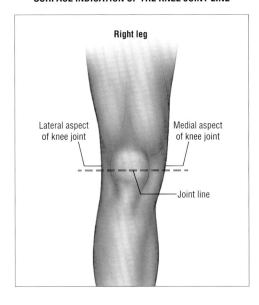

Many patients with knee pain describe their pain as being around the knee-cap or at a point where the hamstring tendons attach (semitendinosus).

BONY ANATOMY OF THE KNEE

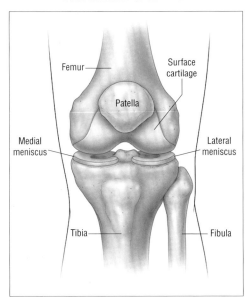

ATTACHMENT OF MUSCLES TO PES ANSERINUS

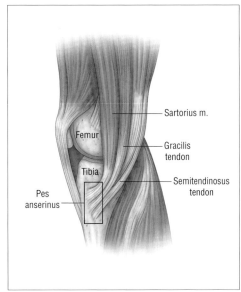

If your pain is not in the proper place, a meniscal tear is not the cause of your pain.

One final indicator of an acute torn meniscus causing knee pain is buckling. If you are walking and intermittently feel that the knee is going to give out, this may be due to a meniscal tear. However, there are other conditions that can cause this, so this is not an automatic indicator of a torn meniscus on its own. But if you are being told that the cause of your knee pain is a torn meniscus and you are not buckling, then that diagnosis should be called into question.

Testing a Meniscal Tear Diagnosis at the Knee: To confirm that the cause of knee pain is due to a meniscal tear, start by checking both the active and passive ranges of motion for your knee.

To test your active range of motion, first move your unaffected knee through its range of motion. See how much you can straighten and bend it. Then try the painful knee. If there is a substantial loss of range of motion in your ability to straighten or bend your painful knee, this shows a loss of active range of motion. Then test your passive range of motion: have someone else try to straighten and bend your painful knee. If the same substantial loss of range of motion is evident passively, this indicates that a meniscal tear could be the cause of your knee pain. During the test, if it feels as if the knee cannot be moved any farther because something is blocking the range, you can take this as another indication of a possible meniscal tear as the cause of your pain. However, if the active range of motion is decreased because of pain, and the passive range of motion is the same or almost the same as the unaffected leg, then a meniscal tear is most likely not the cause of the knee region pain.

Next, you should use palpation to identify the source of the knee pain. If a meniscal tear is the cause, the pain must be experienced at the joint line (space between the thigh bone and the lower leg bone found on either side of the knee). If pressing on this joint line does not elicit pain, this is an indication that a meniscal tear is not the problem.

Another good test is to simply walk around. See if you can cause your knee to buckle. If you can walk around and climb stairs or go from sitting to standing without your knee buckling, this is a good indication that the pain is not from a torn meniscus.

NECROSIS OF THE FEMORAL HEAD (HIP)

This is a fairly rare occurrence at the hip joint. Necrosis of the femoral head is where the blood supply to the head of the thigh bone is damaged or lost and the cartilage and a portion of the bone that makes up the ball portion of the hip joint dies. If this were to occur, there would be a major loss of the structure of the hip joint as there would be substantial damage to the head of the thigh bone. If this happens, you can expect a major loss of range of motion of the hip joint.

Testing a Necrosis of the Femoral Head Diagnosis: If a diagnostic test shows necrosis of the femoral head, this is very likely the cause of your hip pain. However, you can also perform active and passive range-of-motion tests to double-check. To do this, lie on your back on a flat surface and pull the knee on your painful side toward your chest as far as you can. Then have somebody else move your leg for you. This test looks at the range of motion of the knee into hip flexion.

Then you will test the hip's range of motion in abduction. To do this, move the leg associated with your painful hip region out to the side as far as you can go. Then do the test again with somebody else moving your leg.

In both the test for hip flexion and the test for abduction, the movements you make on your own test the active range of motion. Those done by your helper test the passive range of motion.

When trying to move the hip—actively or passively—through its full range of motion, you should reach a point where, in essence, you hit a wall. You would not be able to move beyond this no matter how hard you tried. Another thing to note is that if you have necrosis of the femoral head, you should have difficulty bearing weight because of pain. If these two symptoms are found in addition to the diagnostic test, then surgery is recommended.

NERVE ROOT IMPINGEMENT/PINCHED NERVE (NECK, MID-BACK, LOWER BACK)

This is the diagnosis most people are concerned about getting because it sounds quite serious. It seems so open-and-shut that a nerve root impingement can cause neck and back pain. And if you've had pain at your neck, mid-back, or lower back and a pinched nerve was found, this is likely the diagnosis you received.

The reality is that in most cases, nerve root impingements, or pinched nerves, could not cause pain in any of these regions—or at least not solely in one of these regions. Here's why. Coming off the spinal cord, at every level of the spine, are nerve roots. The nerve roots innervate specific areas of skin called dermatomes to provide sensation. What has to be understood is that the vast majority of the nerve roots that come out of your spine do not innervate areas of skin in the neck or the lower back. The majority of nerve roots that come out of the cervical spine run from the shoulder down to the hand, so a pinched nerve in this cervical spine would lead to altered sensation in the shoulder, arm, or hand. The nerves coming from the thoracic spine run around the torso like thin circles. While they do innervate the mid-back, any pain associated with a pinched thoracic nerve would have to reach all the way around your body, so it cannot be blamed for back pain alone. And the nerves originating in the lumbar region innervate the legs, so a pinched lumbar nerve would cause symptoms in the legs.

DERMATOMAL CHART OF THE BODY

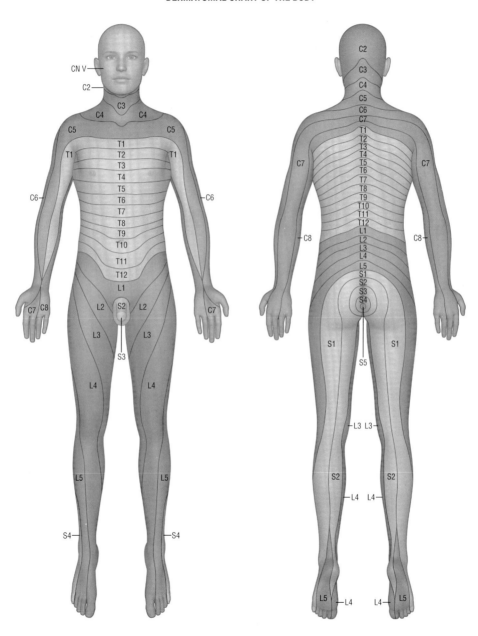

The only time a diagnosis of a pinched nerve causing neck pain makes sense is if the MRI reveals a C3 nerve root impingement. The nerves that come out of this region innervate the skin at the neck, running down the neck, or upper trapezius (trap) region, the area of your neck that connects the neck to the shoulders. However, this is not a common nerve root to be impinged.

If the C3 nerve root is impinged, we would expect that pain would be increased by putting additional pressure on the impinged nerve. The pain would be referred to your neck from the pinched nerve, and thus it would not increase through additional pressure on the neck muscles.

Testing a Nerve Root Impingement Diagnosis at the Neck: In the case of neck pain, other than a possible impingement of the C3 nerve root, there is no test that needs to be done. Nerve root impingement leading to neck pain is not possible except for the C3 nerve root.

If you do get a diagnosis of an impinged C3 nerve root, you should use palpation to determine whether the pain is point-tender or referred. To do this, apply pressure to the C3 vertebra. If this pressure increases the pain, this is a sign that the nerve root impingement could be the cause of your neck pain. If it doesn't, this indicates another source.

SIDE VIEW OF CERVICAL SPINE

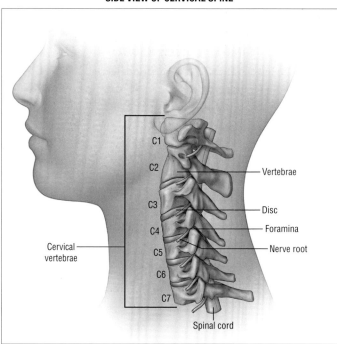

You will also want to apply pressure directly to the area of your neck where you are experiencing the pain. If you palpate the upper trap region away from the spine and pain is elicited, this indicates that the pain being experienced is point-tender, meaning that the pain is not being referred from an impinged nerve root.

Testing a Nerve Root Impingement Diagnosis at the Mid-Back or Lower Back: In the thoracic region, if a nerve root impingement occurred, then the symptom experienced would present as a region of pain that spans the width of that level of the spine and runs around the entire torso. If the pain being experienced is simply in the thoracic spine area, between the shoulder blades, for instance, it is impossible that this symptom resulted from a nerve root impingement. Therefore, no testing is necessary.

The same holds true for the pain in the lower back. There are no lumbar nerve roots that innervate the area of skin at the lower back; therefore, the finding of a nerve root impingement cannot cause pain at the lower back. No test is necessary.

PATELLOFEMORAL SYNDROME/CHONDROMALACIA PATELLAE (KNEE)

This is a very common diagnosis given when a person has pain around the kneecap. The phrase *patellofemoral syndrome* simply means pain at the joint between the kneecap and the thigh bone. One potential cause of patellofemoral syndrome is chondromalacia patella, which is a softening of the cartilage that makes up the back of the kneecap. The implication is that because of this softening, the gliding of the kneecap through the knee joint will cause pain behind the kneecap. But there are many other causes of pain at the joint between the thigh bone and kneecap, so assuming that the cause of the pain is the softening of the cartilage behind the kneecap isn't the best choice to make. Muscles play such an important role in how the kneecap runs through the knee joint that it is much more likely that the pain is coming from a muscular deficit than softening of the cartilage.

Testing a Patellofemoral Syndrome Diagnosis at the Knee: I don't have a test to confirm whether softening of the cartilage behind the kneecap is directly causing pain. Because there are so many other possible causes, I would suggest that you refer to Part II of this book to determine if the cause of the pain is muscular in nature. If not, then the treatments for soft cartilage should be investigated.

PELVIC FRACTURE (GLUTEAL REGION)

A pelvic fracture is often given as the diagnosis for people who have pain in the gluteal region, and, as with many other diagnoses, this is based solely on the finding of a fracture on an X-ray. There are a couple of things to consider when determining whether or not a fracture is the cause of your pain. First, even after a fracture heals, it will show up on an X-ray, so while a fracture can clearly be seen, it is possible that it has been around for a while. With only the X-ray as evidence, it is *assumed* that this fracture happened recently and thus started inciting pain.

Second, this diagnosis often comes because someone falls and then begins feeling gluteal pain. This is what inspires the trip to get a diagnosis in the first place. The combination of a fall and the finding of a fracture on an X-ray is generally what brings about the diagnosis. However, what is rarely considered is that when a person falls, he or she generally tries to stop the fall, thus straining a muscle in this region. Or the impact of the fall may have been on the muscle rather than the bone, and thus he or she is suffering from a contusion of the muscle. So the important thing to note when trying to diagnose if a pelvic fracture is actually the cause of your gluteal pain is the location of the pain itself.

For a pelvic fracture to be the true cause of your pain, the pain must be experienced on the pelvic bones. If your pain is not where the bones are, then the pain is not coming from the identified pelvic fracture. If the pain is in the gluteal region itself, where the majority of the region is filled with muscle, the pelvic fracture is most likely not the source of your pain.

ANATOMY OF THE PELVIS

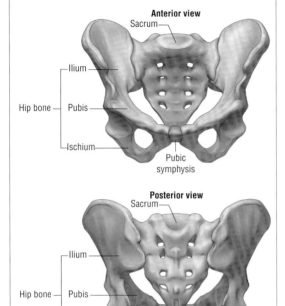

Anterior view

Sacrum

Ilium

Hip bone — Pubis

Ischium

Pubic symphysis

Posterior view

Sacrum

Ilium

Hip bone — Pubis

Ischium

Coccyx

HIP MUSCULATURE

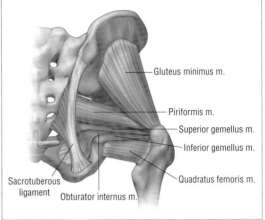

Gluteus minimus m.

Piriformis m.

Superior gemellus m.

Inferior gemellus m.

Quadratus femoris m.

Sacrotuberous ligament

Obturator internus m.

Testing a Pelvic Fracture Diagnosis in the Gluteal Region: If you have fallen—or experienced another trauma that put excessive force on your pelvic bone—and you are experiencing pain in your gluteal region that wasn't there before, it's important that you do get an X-ray. In this instance, if an X-ray identifies a pelvic fracture, there is a good chance that your pain is the result of the fracture and you should wait for it to heal. This will take a few weeks, but the pain should resolve within a reasonable amount of time after that. However, if your pain continues for several months, the cause is either that the fracture is not healing properly, which is unusual, or the pain was not due to the pelvic fracture.

The simplest test to do to check whether a pelvic fracture is the cause of your pain is palpation. The gluteal region is generally composed of muscle, except at the top and at the center where the buttocks meet. Differentiating the pelvis from the muscles in this region is key to figuring out if the pain is coming from the fracture. A fracture will not refer pain, and therefore the pain being experienced from a fracture must be experienced where the fracture occurred. So to test this diagnosis, you will press on the location of the fracture on the bone itself. If the pain is being experienced elsewhere in the region, the diagnosis of pain from a fracture is incorrect.

ROTATOR CUFF TEAR (SHOULDER)

Finding a torn rotator cuff through the use of an MRI is extremely common. But just like diagnoses of arthritis, stenosis, meniscal tears, and herniated discs, a rotator cuff tear, unless associated with trauma, is most likely a progressive degenerative change that occurs so slowly that the body doesn't even create a pain signal to identify that the change is occurring.

To understand the possibility of a rotator cuff tear as the cause of your pain, you first have to understand what the rotator cuff is and how it interacts with your shoulder joint. The rotator cuff consists of four muscles that attach from the shoulder blade to the upper arm bone. Its purpose is both to keep the arm bone in the shoulder joint with maximum congruency between the bones and to depress (pull down) the head of the upper arm bone in the shoulder joint while the arm is raised. If there were a tear of the rotator cuff, then the head of the upper arm bone would not be pulled down during shoulder motion. This would cause the head of the upper arm bone to rise and impact the acromion process, the bone at the top of the shoulder joint. This would alter the mechanics of the shoulder, making raising the arm impossible. Active range of motion would be severely decreased—you would likely only be able to raise your arm about 110 degrees (just slightly above shoulder height) rather than the normal 180 degrees (up to your ear).

An acute rotator cuff tear, in most cases, is associated with a traumatic event. You will have full range of motion of the shoulder joint before the trauma, but afterward it will be severely reduced. Remember that this loss of range of motion is not associated with pain. It is associated with the altered mechanics of the shoulder because the torn rotator cuff is not allowing for normal movement of the head of the upper arm bone in the shoulder joint.

Testing a Rotator Cuff Tear Diagnosis at the Shoulder: To test the validity of a rotator cuff tear diagnosis as the cause of your pain, the first thing to do is think about how the pain came about. Did you experience some sort of trauma that incited the pain? Or did the pain slowly come on without any excessive force applied to the shoulder region? If the answer to the second question is yes—you don't remember a trauma—it is unlikely that a rotator cuff tear is the cause of your shoulder pain.

You should also complete a range-of-motion test. To do this, raise the arm overhead both in front of you and to the side. See how far you can raise it. If there isn't a major loss of range of motion, there is a good chance that the cause of the pain is not from a rotator cuff tear. You can double-check this finding by doing a passive range-of-motion test for the shoulder. Because there is no alteration to the structural integrity of the shoulder joint, having somebody else raise your arm in front and to the side of you will show that you have full or almost completely full range of motion.

RUPTURED DISC (NECK, MID-BACK, LOWER BACK)

A ruptured disc is the most severe variation you might find in problems associated with the vertebral discs of the spine. To understand what a ruptured disc is, you'll need to understand the structure of the spine. The spine is composed of spinal cord protected by 29 vertebrae; all but the sacral vertebrae are separated by a disc that has a gel-like substance called the nucleus pulposus in its center. The gel is surrounded by a connective tissue covering called the annulus. The gel is designed to take the force of gravity pushing down on you and your spine. And the annulus is designed to keep the gel in place in the center of the disc. When a person has bad posture due to muscle weakness or imbalances, the forces on the spine can be altered and the force of gravity pressing down on the individual and his or her spine may not be centered. This can cause excessive forces to develop on one side of the spine or the other. These excessive forces can push the gel outside the annulus. In some cases, malformation of the disc can be responsible for causing a shift of the gel toward the side that forces it outside of the annulus covering. In some cases, a severe trauma can play a role in creating a ruptured disc.

This is now a very dangerous situation. The gel can enter the spinal column and impact not just the nerve roots (as in the case of the herniated disc) but also the spinal cord.

If you have a ruptured disc, the symptoms would be severe and could include extreme weakness or paralysis, loss of your bowel and bladder function, or altered sensation of large portions of your limbs. It is important to understand that simple neck or back pain is certainly not the type of symptom you would expect with a ruptured disc. The symptoms would be much more widespread and severe.

Testing a Ruptured Disc Diagnosis at the Neck, Mid-Back, or Lower Back: The finding of a ruptured disc should not be considered as the cause of pain as a general rule. The effects of a ruptured disc would be much more widespread and severe; thus, no test is required.

SCOLIOSIS (MID-BACK, LOWER BACK)

Scoliosis is one of the most misdiagnosed causes of back pain for both the mid-back and the lower back. Scoliosis simply means a curvature of the spine, which means that the spinal components are not lining up over one another in a normal position. There is no variation to the structure of the vertebrae with scoliosis—the vertebrae are completely intact.

NORMAL SPINE AND SCOLIOTIC SPINE

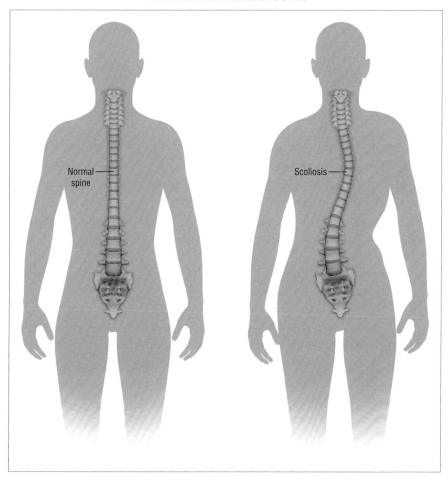

Normal
spine

Scoliosis

Scoliosis can be broken down into two types: structural and functional. Structural scoliosis is the type that develops during growth, starting at an early age. As the person grows, the spine does not develop normally and ends up having a curvature to it. This is a permanent change in structure, and the curve in the spine is more apt to be severe. In functional scoliosis, the curvature of the spine is caused by a muscle imbalance between the muscles on either side of the spine. This can develop when a person is an adult, and since most people have one side that is stronger than the other, many people develop scoliosis.

In the majority of cases, the pain that is generally associated with scoliosis is due to a muscle imbalance between the muscles on either side of the spine. The only difference between this imbalance in structural versus functional scoliosis is that in functional scoliosis, the scoliosis is a dual symptom that can be resolved by strength training.

In the muscle imbalance in scoliosis, the muscles on the stronger side of the back tend to shorten. They can shorten enough to strain and emit pain at their connection to the spine. Alternatively, the muscles on the opposite side of the spine can become overstretched and lose their ability to create force, causing them to strain and emit pain at their attachment to the spine. In either case, although the pain appears to be experienced at the spine, it is not the vertebrae that are emitting the pain signal; it is the muscles that are attaching to the spine.

The only way that scoliosis can cause pain is if the curvature is so great that the vertebrae have been compressed on one side and are experiencing fracturing. The only cure for this type of damage is surgery.

Testing a Scoliosis Diagnosis at the Mid-Back or Lower Back: While it isn't imperative to know, you may be interested to see if your scoliosis is functional or structural. To do this, simply stand up straight and have somebody look at your back. Then bend forward. If your spine straightens out when you bend forward, the scoliosis is functional and can be improved with resolution of the muscle imbalance creating the curvature. If the curvature doesn't disappear when you bend forward, then your scoliosis is structural and most likely cannot be altered. However, this still does not mean that it is the cause of your pain.

The key to testing for pain from scoliosis is to see whether the tissue emitting the pain is the vertebrae or the muscle that attaches to the vertebrae. Palpation, or feeling the tissues, can assist in this process.

At the level of your back where you are experiencing pain, press just to the side of the vertebrae and feel the attachment of the muscles to the vertebrae. If pain is experienced, this reinforces the idea that the pain is actually being emitted from the muscle, not the spine. Then press on the vertebra itself to see if this increases your pain. If not, this disputes the claim that scoliosis is the cause of your pain. The goal is to determine whether it is the muscle attaching to the spine or the spine itself emitting the pain.

If the pain is in your lower back, in addition to palpation, you'll want to look at your posture and ability to move after sitting. The hip flexor muscles attach to the five lumbar vertebrae, and these can also cause lower back pain. One possible clue to determining whether the cause of the pain is from the vertebrae or the hip flexor muscles is whether you are having difficulty standing upright. This indicates that the hip flexors are shortened and strained, emitting pain at their attachment to the lumbar spine. The other functional clue is difficulty in standing up after sitting for a while. The seated position is an opportunity for the hip flexors to shorten, so when you try to stand up, it is difficult for the muscles to lengthen again, which is required for standing upright. If the hip flexors are found to be emitting the pain, versus pain coming from the spine, this confirms that scoliosis is not the cause of your pain.

SI JOINT DYSFUNCTION (GLUTEAL REGION)

I consider this the granddaddy of all structural diagnoses for gluteal region pain. In fact, when pain exists in the gluteal region, many medical specialists immediately look to the SI joint as the catchall answer for the cause of pain. Typically the diagnosis is made when an arthritic change is found at the joint through an X-ray.

The SI (sacroiliac) joint is between the sacral spine and the pelvis. Movement occurs at this joint with hip motions, such as bending and straightening, and moving the leg out to the side and back in. However, this joint doesn't allow for much motion because it is very shallow and composed of two long flat bones versus the typical ball-and-socket joint.

SACROILIAC JOINT

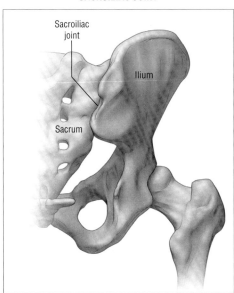

Sacroiliac
joint

Ilium

Sacrum

Because of the common finding of arthritic changes at this joint, it's understandable why any detection of arthritis would be blamed for pain. However, just as with arthritis, the important thing to understand is whether the joint has been compromised enough to cause pain. This would be indicated by reduced range of motion. Also remember that the piriformis muscle, which starts at the sacral spine bones and attaches to the hip joint, passes the SI joint. It is important to be able to differentiate whether pain is coming from the SI joint or the piriformis muscle.

Testing an SI Joint Dysfunction Diagnosis in the Gluteal Region: To test the SI joint dysfunction diagnosis, the first thing you need to do is check the range of motion of the SI joint, which you do by testing hip flexion (bending your hip) and abduction (moving your leg out). With hip flexion, the pelvic portion of the SI joint moves on the sacral portion of the SI joint. The pelvic portion rotates forward. With hip abduction, the SI joint surfaces approximate one another—they move closer together.

A simple test to check the integrity of the SI joint is to perform hip flexion and hip abduction. To do this, stand and hold on to a sturdy surface to balance yourself. First, raise the knee of the unaffected leg toward the chest as high as you can, and then return it to the start position. Then move it out to the side as far as you can, and then return it to the start position again. Next, perform the same two movements with the affected side. If there is a difference in range of motion and there is a correlative experience of pain at the SI joint on the side with the limited range of motion, then this is a positive test for SI joint dysfunction. If there is no difference in range of motion of either leg, then there is no reason to believe that the SI joint is the cause of the gluteal region pain.

The second test to do is palpation of both the joint itself and the piriformis muscle, which attaches to the sacral spine and passes by the SI joint on its way across the gluteal region to the hip joint. The SI joint is fairly easy to identify by feeling for it. Press on the joint or have somebody press on it for you. The SI joint can be found close to the top of the buttocks, just a couple of inches on either side of the spine. Try to find the space between the sacral spine and the pelvis. If pressing directly on the joint increases your pain, then this is a positive sign that the SI joint is the cause of your pain.

SPINE AND PELVIS

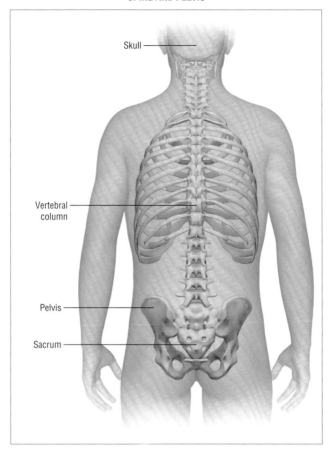

Now examine the piriformis muscle. Palpate this muscle along its path from the sacral spine diagonally across the gluteal region to the hip joint. If the SI joint is causing your pain, this palpation should not increase the level of pain you are experiencing. Palpating the SI joint and the piriformis muscle should help you understand which of these tissues is emitting the pain signal in the gluteal region.

PIRIFORMIS ATTACHMENT NEAR THE SI JOINT

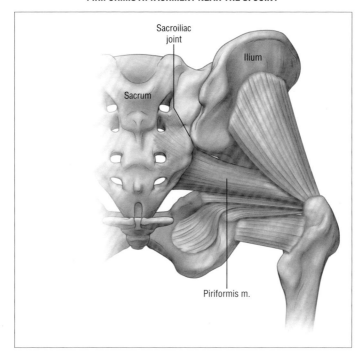

SPINAL FRACTURE (GLUTEAL REGION)

The part of the spine that is associated with the gluteal region is the sacral spine. The sacral spine lies below the lumbar spine and consists of five fused bones. There are no intervertebral discs located between the vertebrae. Just as with the lumbar spine, a spinal fracture is possible, but it is less likely in this region. Typically a spinal fracture in the sacral spine is going to be seen with a significant trauma.

In this instance of a fracture being the cause of pain, pain would be experienced only at the level of the fracture. Pain across a wide area of the gluteal region cannot be caused by a fracture of a sacral spine vertebra.

Testing a Spinal Fracture Diagnosis in the Gluteal Region: If you are experiencing pain in a small area associated with the sacral spine, you'll want to determine whether the pain is coming from the fracture or an adjacent tissue to the spine. You can do this by using palpation. A fracture should only create pain at the location of the fracture, while a strained muscle will cause pain away from the vertebra. When pressing on the center of the sacral vertebrae, see if the pain is elicited at that point or along the edges of the spine where the piriformis muscles attach. You can also try to feel the piriformis muscle as it moves from the sacral spine along its path across the gluteal region to the hip joint. If pain continues to be elicited as the piriformis is palpated, it is more likely that the muscle is the cause of the pain versus the vertebrae.

THE SPINE

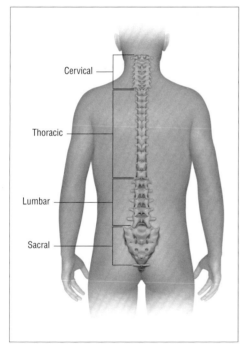

Cervical

Thoracic

Lumbar

Sacral

PIRIFORMIS ATTACHMENT NEAR SI JOINT

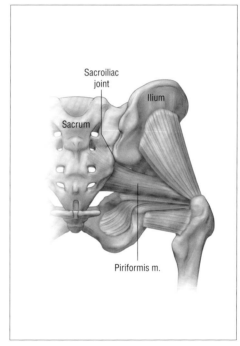

Sacroiliac joint

Ilium

Sacrum

Piriformis m.

SPONDYLOLISTHESIS (NECK, LOWER BACK)

This is a scary-sounding word, but it simply means a shifting of the vertebrae from front to back. The spinal column is held in place by several ligaments and connective tissue structures. The goal is to keep the vertebrae in proper alignment because the spinal column encases the spinal cord. If a vertebra were to become free from the ligaments and connective tissue that support it, it could shift freely. There are degrees that the vertebrae can shift forward and back, and the greater the shift, the more potential there is that the spinal cord will be impinged on and a symptom created. It is important to understand that this diagnosis does not imply that there is any structural alteration to the vertebrae such as a fracture, simply that it is free to shift. Since there is not a structural alteration, there is no reason to think that the vertebrae would emit a pain signal. And if the vertebrae were to shift significantly enough on the spinal cord, this would create substantial symptoms, such as bowel and bladder dysfunction or paralysis. Neck or back pain would certainly not be a symptom of a shifting vertebra that impacts the spinal cord.

Testing a Spondylolisthesis Diagnosis at the Neck or Lower Back: The finding of spondylolisthesis should not be considered the cause of pain as a general rule. The effects of this would be much more widespread and severe; thus, no test is required.

SPONDYLOSIS (NECK, LOWER BACK)

Again, this sounds ominous, but spondylosis simply means arthritis of the spine. This diagnosis could likely be given to anybody over the age of 60—whether they have pain or not. It's just so common. But just like arthritis, which I described at the beginning of this chapter, structural variations from this form of osteoarthritis take years to occur. The progression is so slow that it doesn't generally ignite a pain signal. The only time arthritis can become a factor in creating pain is when the arthritic change overtakes the joint space between the vertebrae. When this happens, free motion of the vertebrae is prohibited, and the vertebrae rub against one another, creating irritation and pain.

Testing a Spondylosis Diagnosis at the Neck: The way to determine whether an arthritic change has reached the point where it can cause neck pain is to look at the ability of the vertebrae of the cervical spine to glide. When you turn your head or look up and down, the vertebrae of the spine shift on one another. This action occurs automatically.

To test to see if the vertebrae of the neck are able to glide freely requires somebody to move your neck for you. To do this test, simply lie down on your back and have somebody cradle your head in their hands. Have the person try to move your head from side to side and then up and down without your bending or rotating at the neck.

ANTERIOR/POSTERIOR GLIDES—START

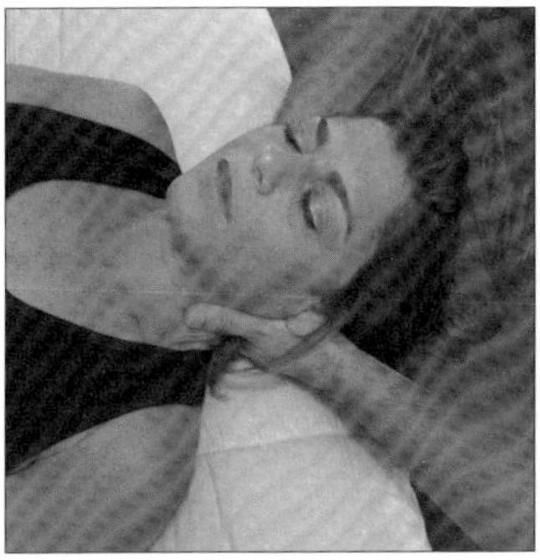

ANTERIOR/POSTERIOR GLIDES—FINISH

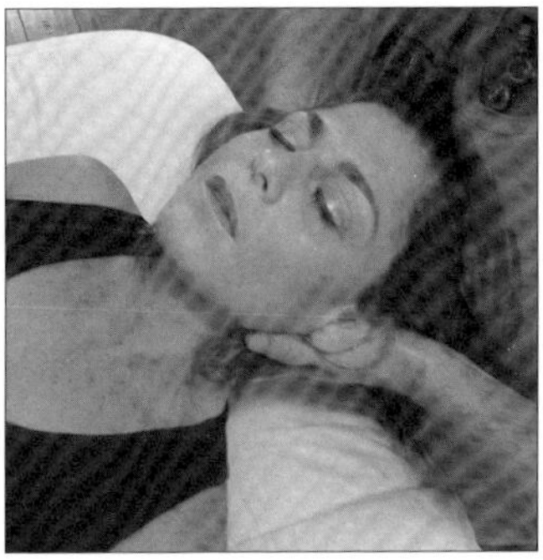

LATERAL GLIDES—START

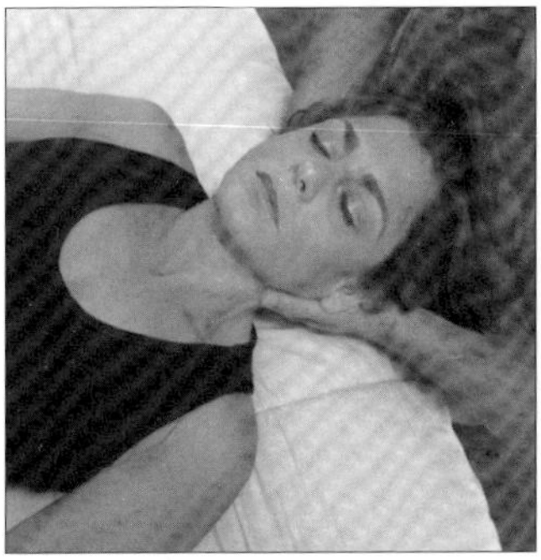

LATERAL GLIDES—ONE SIDE

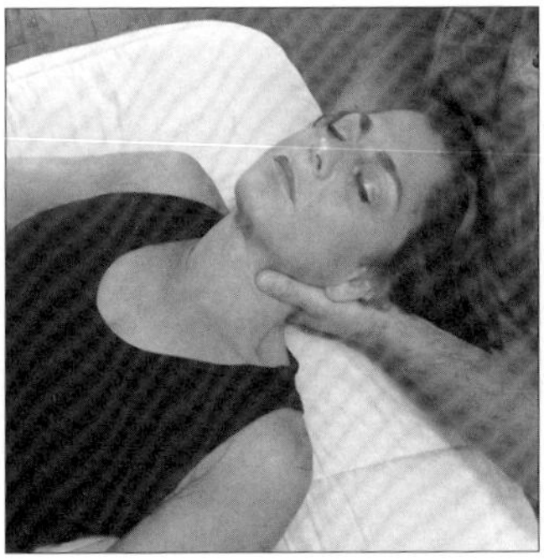

LATERAL GLIDES—OTHER SIDE

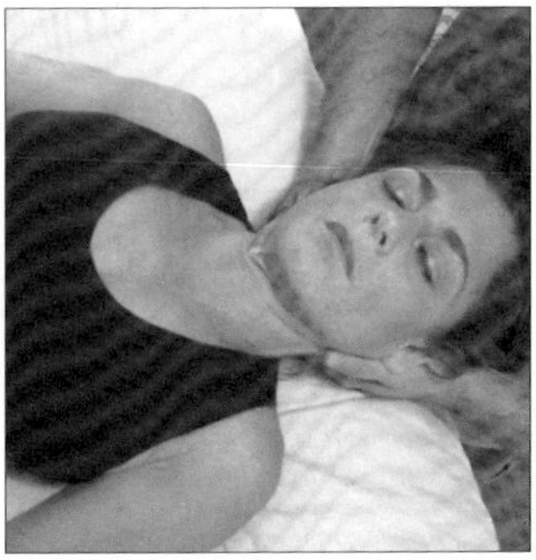

If your head can shift in both of these directions, there is free motion between the vertebrae, meaning that the arthritic change is minimal and is most likely not causing your neck pain. If there is a blockage or inability to glide the vertebrae, then there is a good chance the arthritic change is a factor in the neck pain.

Testing a Spondylosis Diagnosis at the Lower Back: There is a much higher risk of osteoarthritis developing in the neck versus the lumbar spine because the neck is where much more motion occurs. The lower back has minimal rotation and side bending occurring since most movement at the lower back is performed bending forward and back. In addition, it is mostly used as a way of transmitting the weight of the torso and upper body to the ground as well as stabilizing the torso to allow for activities to be performed by the arms and legs.

The one possible cause of osteoarthritis at the lumbar spine being severe enough to create pain and limit movement is a disease entity called ankylosing spondylitis. This can be identified by X-ray and typically begins by affecting the SI joints and lumbar spine.

As a general rule, osteoarthritis is not going to cause pain at the lumbar spine, and therefore no clinical test is available to differentiate it as a cause of pain.

STENOSIS (NECK, MID-BACK, LOWER BACK)

While *stenosis* sounds dangerous and imposing, it simply means narrowing, and the theory of stenosis causing pain is basically the same as the theory of a herniated disc causing pain. In both cases, pain is attributed to an impacted nerve root. If stenosis of the spinal cord were to occur, then you would expect the symptoms to be much greater than isolated pain in the region of the neck, mid-back, or lower back. So let's go back to my explanation of a nerve root impingement to understand why a compressed nerve root would not cause neck or back pain.

Coming off the spinal cord, at every level of the spine, are nerve roots. The nerve roots innervate specific areas of skin called dermatomes to provide sensation. What has to be understood is that the vast majority of the nerve roots that come out of your spine do not innervate areas of skin in the neck or the lower back. The majority of nerve roots that come out of the cervical spine run from the shoulder down to the hand, so a pinched nerve in the cervical spine would lead to altered sensation in the shoulder, arm, or hand. The nerves coming from the thoracic spine run around the torso like thin circles. While they do innervate the mid-back, any pain associated with a pinched thoracic nerve would have to reach all the way around your body, so it cannot be blamed for back pain alone. And the nerves originating in the lumbar region innervate the legs, so a pinched lumbar nerve would cause symptoms in the legs.

DERMATOMAL CHART OF THE BODY

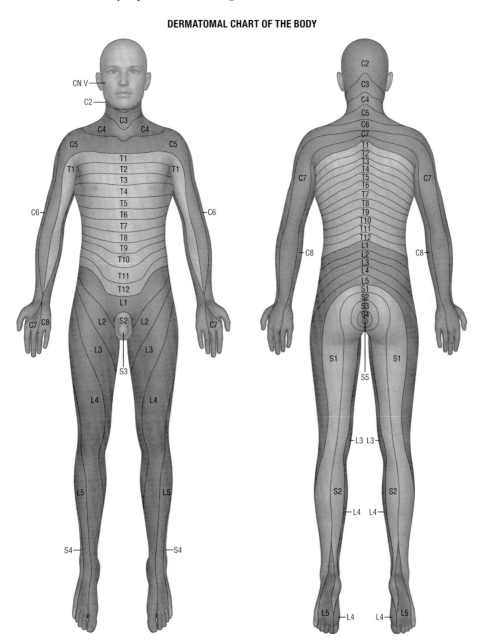

With stenosis, the compression of the nerve root is due to the narrowing of the foramen (the opening at the spinal column where each nerve root leaves the spinal cord). The cause of the narrowing can be related to different types of disc disease, such as bulging or herniated discs and degenerative disc disease.

Testing a Stenosis Diagnosis at the Neck, Mid-Back, or Lower Back: The key to knowing if stenosis is causing your pain is understanding just how the nerves work. The nerve roots innervate specific areas of skin called dermatomes to provide sensation. If an impinged nerve root from stenosis is the cause of your symptoms, the symptom must be in the area of skin innervated by the nerve root. It must be within the area and nowhere else. So you must assess if the pain you are experiencing is in the proper place based on where the stenosis was identified. You can do this by using the chart on the previous page to see where on the body the nerves associated with your stenosis innervate. If the pain is outside that area, the diagnosis that stenosis is the cause of your pain is likely incorrect.

When testing whether stenosis is the cause of pain, notice whether the pain is referred or point-tender. In the case of stenosis, you will use palpation by pressing in the area where you feel pain. If the pain increases, this is a sign that the pain is point-tender and not coming from stenosis. If the pain does not increase, this implies that the pain is referred, and this corroborates the diagnosis of stenosis.

THE IMPORTANCE OF TESTING YOUR DIAGNOSIS

I have treated so many people who have come to me after being misdiagnosed through the use of an MRI or X-ray. They have been treated with drugs. They have gone through unnecessary surgeries. They have done so many things to address their pain, and yet still they've found no relief. It is heartbreaking. And this is why it's so important to make sure the diagnosis you are given matches the symptoms you are experiencing.

One of my most memorable cases of someone suffering from a misdiagnosis was a patient I treated who had surgery for a meniscal tear. He had knee pain, and an MRI had shown a meniscal tear. He had chosen me to perform post-surgery physical therapy because I had successfully treated his wife for gluteal region pain after she was misdiagnosed with stenosis of the lumbar spine. Since he'd had the surgery already, there was nothing I could do except treat him for the postsurgical symptoms: swelling, pain at the surgery site, and decreased strength of muscles associated with the knee. Within a couple of weeks, these symptoms resolved, but the man continued to complain about the same pain he'd had before the surgery. A simple evaluation using the tests I describe in Part II of this book determined that his pain was coming from the attachment of the medial hamstring tendon that attaches near the knee.

I asked him if he would allow me to treat him using this new diagnosis, and he said that he didn't care what the treatment was—he just wanted the pain resolved and his life back. After two weeks of simple muscle exercises, his pain was gone and he had full function in his knee. He was able to return to golf, which was his passion. A few months later, he came in to tell me just how happy he was. He also told me about a follow-up visit with the surgeon during which he told the surgeon about how after surgery his pain was exactly the same but after I treated him for a hamstring strain his pain was fully resolved. He was angry and asked the surgeon if he had really needed the surgery for the meniscal tear. The surgeon answered, "Maybe you did, maybe you didn't. I guess we will never know." Can you imagine?

So please, take this as a wake-up call. Please evaluate whether or not the diagnosis you are given makes sense. *Never accept a diagnosis simply based on an MRI or X-ray.* The information in this chapter helps you determine whether or not a diagnosis is valid. You can only be satisfied with a diagnosis when it goes one step further: when it determines through clinical testing which tissue is emitting the pain signal as well as which tissues are not emitting the pain signal. This step further is what I'll teach you how to do in the next part of this book.

PART II

RESOLVING
PAIN

CHAPTER 5

THE
NECK

MUSCULATURE OF THE NECK AND UPPER BACK

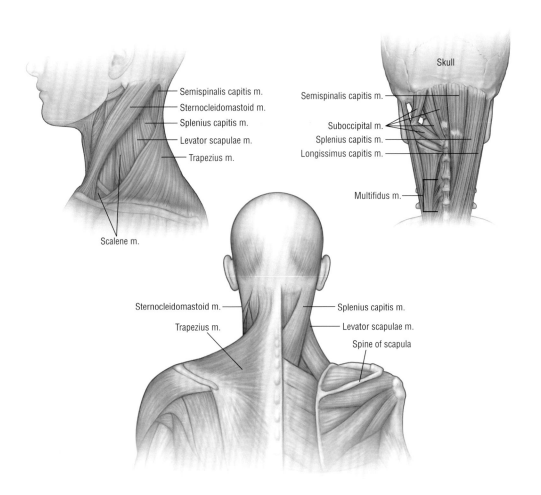

Semispinalis capitis m.
Sternocleidomastoid m.
Splenius capitis m.
Levator scapulae m.
Trapezius m.

Scalene m.

Skull

Semispinalis capitis m.

Suboccipital m.
Splenius capitis m.
Longissimus capitis m.

Multifidus m.

Sternocleidomastoid m.

Trapezius m.

Splenius capitis m.

Levator scapulae m.

Spine of scapula

In this chapter you will find a description of the muscle groups possibly involved in creating pain in your neck, along with clinical tests to confirm which muscle is emitting the pain. Once you have determined where the pain is coming from, please go to the Appendix to learn the muscle-strengthening exercises that will help resolve your pain.

PAIN ON BOTH SIDES OF THE NECK

If you have pain across your neck—not simply on one side—you will likely find that the cause is an imbalance in strength between the muscles in the front of your body and the muscles in the back of the body. In the front of your body this involves the pecs (chest muscles), anterior deltoids (front shoulder muscles), and biceps (front upper arm muscles), and in the back you have the middle trapezius, or mid-traps, and rhomboids (the muscles between the shoulder blades), posterior deltoids (back shoulder muscles), and triceps (back upper arm muscles). As a general rule, the muscles in the front of your body are stronger than those in the back of your body because most activities are performed in front of the body—thus the front-of-body muscles are worked more regularly.

If the imbalance between these muscle groups increases significantly enough, the muscles in the back are no longer able to act as a counterforce to the muscles in the front and the shoulders pull forward, creating an improper posture known as forward shoulder posture. In this posture, the shoulder blades are pulled outward, away from the spine, and any muscle that attaches to the shoulder blade from the skull or spine becomes overstretched.

In the case of forward shoulder posture, the levator scapulae (muscles that run from the upper edge of the shoulder blade to the upper cervical spine) become overstretched. When muscles become overstretched, they lose their ability to create force, and, in this instance, that means that the levator scapulae cannot adequately support the head. This leads to a posture known as forward head posture. Owing to the strain of the levator scapulae, the muscles emit pain.

Pain may be experienced at any point along the length of the levator scapulae muscle—in the upper cervical region where the muscles attach to the cervical spine, along the length of the neck, or at the upper inner borders of the shoulder blades.

To verify that your pain is coming from strained levator scapulae, you will perform a number of clinical tests, including a posture analysis, palpation, and muscle testing.

Posture Analysis: First, let's look at your posture. As I mentioned, people with pain across the whole neck often have forward head posture. To confirm whether or not you have this posture, have somebody take a full-length photo of you from the side. Simply stand how you would comfortably and normally stand.

Once you have the photo, look at the position of your ear in relationship to your shoulder. If your ear lines up in front of the shoulder when looking at yourself from the side, that describes forward head posture. To determine if you also have forward shoulder posture, look at your shoulder in respect to your hip, knee, and ankle. These joints should roughly align. If the shoulder is in front of hip, knee, and ankle, you have forward shoulder posture. If this posture has reached a more severe extent, you might find a hunching occurring at the lower portion of the cervical spine. This occurs in older people and is often associated with aging; however, this is not simply a result of aging. The muscle imbalance between the front and back muscles has simply become severe. If this improper posture is found, you now have a corroborating finding that your neck pain is the result of the muscle imbalance described.

Palpation: Now let's do some palpation, or the touching of tissues. This is the hardest test to do because you have to identify and press on certain muscles.

To begin this test, simply touch the region of the neck where you are experiencing pain. Press on your neck in various places in an attempt to make your pain worse. Our goal here is to ignite the pain signal, so you can see which muscle is causing the pain. With most people who experience pain across the entire neck, pressing anywhere along the length of the levator scapulae will increase pain. If this is true for you, you now have yet another corroborating finding that the cause of your pain is the muscle imbalance described. Remember, if the pain were coming from a structural variation, such as a herniated disc, stenosis, or a nerve root impingement, pain would only be increased by putting pressure on the structure itself. This would be referred pain. If pain is point-tender, coming from the muscle itself, this is not structural.

Another set of muscles to palpate to confirm whether the cause of the neck pain is a muscle imbalance is the pecs (chest muscles). These muscles attach to the upper arm at the shoulder joint. Just before the pec muscle reaches the shoulder it becomes a tendon. Palpate the chest region just inside the shoulder joint. If tenderness is experienced in this location, this is another corroborating finding that points to a muscle imbalance.

Muscle Testing: Finally, muscle testing can be performed to see if there is a muscle imbalance between the chest muscles and muscles between the shoulder blades. This test requires help from someone else. Simply bend your elbow to 90 degrees with the elbow to the side and raised so it is at shoulder height with your palm facing the floor. Your arm should be parallel to the floor.

MUSCLE TEST—ANTERIOR TORSO MUSCLES

MUSCLE TEST—POSTERIOR TORSO MUSCLES

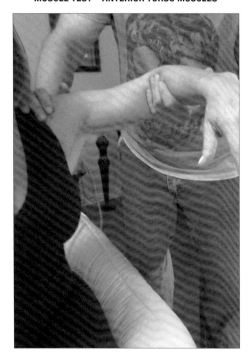
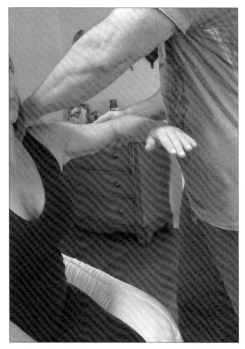

Your helper will be testing how forcefully you are able to resist him or her—both while you are pushing backward and while you are pushing forward. First, you will test your forward strength by having your helper place one hand on the back of your shoulder and the other inside the bend of your elbow. Press your arm forward as powerfully as you can while your helper resists. Next, have him or her put one hand on the front of your shoulder and one on the back of your elbow. Press your arm backward as powerfully as you can while your helper resists. If it is much harder for him or her to resist the forward press than the backward press, you have confirmed that a muscle imbalance exists between the pecs and the muscles between the shoulder blades.

If you have performed all these tests and found positive results, you have confirmation that the cause of your neck pain is a muscle imbalance. The great thing about this is that it is likely that your pain can not only be resolved but also prevented from recurring. I do, however, want to make a brief point here about the severity of the symptoms and the muscle imbalance that might exist. For a good percentage of the people suffering from neck pain due to this muscle imbalance, correctly performing the following strengthening exercises from the Appendix will heal the pain:

1. Posterior Deltoids (page 237)

2. Lat Pulldown with Neutral Bar or Elastic Band (page 235)

3. Skull Crushers (page 239)

4. Lower Trap Exercise (page 236)

For some people, however, the strain of the levator scapulae and pecs may be so severe that thickening developed in the muscle. If this has happened, you may require massage to initially break up the knotting of the muscles. Without doing this, it might be too painful to perform the strengthening exercises and strength will not develop properly, sustaining the imbalance and improper posture. If you're not seeing any improvement after a couple of weeks of training, seek the help of a medical professional skilled in the art of breaking up knots in muscle. This will be key to resolving your pain and achieving full functional capacity.

Keep in mind also that the time frame for correcting this muscle imbalance and resolving your neck pain varies from person to person. Factors such as how long you've had the pain, the severity of the imbalance, your general health, and your level of activity all make a difference. The thing you have to keep in mind is the concept of progress. If your pain level was measured at a 10 out of 10 to start with and then a week later it is a 9 or an 8, then all is well—you are progressing. Try to be realistic about your progress when attempting to resolve your pain. If the pain diminishes in intensity, even if it is a little bit at a time, you know that you're going in the right direction. Conversely, if you are seeing no change in your pain, the validity of what you're doing to resolve it must be questioned. Don't continue to do something if no change occurs.

I would also like to mention that there are a number of things you can do to aid in faster healing and prevent recurrence of pain in both sides of the neck—all of which have to do with your everyday activities. For those people who sit at a computer for large portions of their days, there are a few changes that can make a world of difference to your neck.

1. Raise the monitor so that its center line (from top to bottom) is in line with your eyes, so you're not looking down. Looking down forces the head to move forward and puts greater load on the levator scapulae. Looking forward keeps the head over the spine, causing the spine, rather than the levator scapulae, to support it.

2. Get some support for your forearms when typing. If your arms are allowed to simply hang, the weight pulls on your shoulders and shoulder blades, causing the levator scapulae and other supporting muscles to work harder. If your forearms are supported, the load is eliminated.

3. When sitting in your chair, do not hunch forward. Set the chair so the back is slightly angled back, putting your shoulders ever so slightly behind your hips. This again reinforces a position where the head will be supported by the spine and not the levator scapulae.

Assuming better posture can also be done with activities like driving. Setting the driver's seat so it is slightly angled back, putting your shoulders slightly behind your hips, will cause the spine to support the head more than the levator scapulae.

These techniques will help minimize the forces that can play a role in overworking the levator scapulae, but they should not be done in lieu of resolving the muscle imbalance through proper strength training.

SINGLE-SIDED NECK PAIN

If you have pain on only one side of your neck, you'll want to look to a problem with your shoulder and shoulder blade as a likely cause. This is because muscles like the levator scapulae have a dual function: to support the head and to keep the shoulder blade against the rib cage to allow for normal shoulder function.

The shoulder joint is composed of the upper arm bone and the end of the shoulder blade. When the shoulder joint is moved, the shoulder blade glides on the rib cage. There are a few muscles that are responsible for this—some of the muscles help move it, while others work to keep it pressed tight to the rib cage to allow for the gliding motion. For the shoulder joint to move correctly, these muscles—the stabilizing muscles and the moving muscles—must work together.

Since the levator scapulae, which runs from the shoulder blade to the upper cervical spine, has two roles—both stabilizing the shoulder and supporting the head—it is highly susceptible to straining and causing neck pain. The key thing to remember is that the levator scapulae is typically only susceptible to straining if another muscle has strained first. In the case of shoulder function, it is typically due to a rotator cuff strain. The rotator cuff is one of the key muscle groups involved in shoulder motion and function. It is responsible for keeping the upper portion of the upper arm bone in the shoulder joint.

I would like to be clear that I am describing a rotator cuff strain, not a tear. In most cases the rotator cuff strains only because one of the muscles holding the shoulder blade against the rib cage has strained as well. A strain in the serratus anterior, rhomboids, or mid-traps leads to an instability of the shoulder blade against the rib cage. In turn, the rotator cuff has to work harder to keep the upper arm bone in the shoulder joint. The excess load caused by the lack of stability is enough to cause the rotator cuff to strain. Once this strains, then the levator scapulae is often the next to go.

To verify that your neck pain is coming from a strained levator scapulae, you will perform a number of clinical tests, including an analysis of the location of your pain, palpation, muscle testing, and flexibility testing.

Location of Your Symptoms: A possible sign that the cause is muscular is if you are experiencing pain in both your neck and your shoulder-blade region on the same side. It is certainly possible that the levator scapulae and the rotator cuff could be emitting pain at these two areas. Because these two muscle groups work so closely together, this is a clear sign that the cause is muscular.

Palpation: Now let's do some palpation, or the touching of tissues. This is the hardest test to do because you have to identify and press on certain muscles.

Remember the goal of palpation is to ignite the pain signal, so we can see which muscle is causing the pain. With most people who experience pain on one side of the neck, pressing on the levator scapulae where it attaches to the upper inner border of the shoulder blade provides a substantial increase in pain. If this is true for you, you now have yet another corroborating finding that the cause of your pain is a problem in the shoulder or shoulder joint.

You can also press on the rotator cuff muscle called the infraspinatus to see if it is knotted and strained. This will show that a problem in the rotator cuff is likely leading to a problem in the levator scapulae.

Remember, if the pain were coming from a structural variation, such as a herniated disc, stenosis, or a nerve root impingement, pain would only be increased by putting pressure on the structure itself. This would be referred pain. If pain is point-tender, coming from the muscle itself, this is not structural.

Muscle Testing: Muscle testing the rotator cuff will help confirm that the levator scapulae has strained as a result of a loss of shoulder function from the strain of other muscles. To muscle test the rotator cuff, you will need someone to help you. On the unaffected side, keeping the top of your arm flush against your body, bend your elbow to 90 degrees. Your forearm will be facing forward and your hand will be thumb side up, as if you're positioning it to shake hands with someone. Next, have your helper place one hand on the outside of your elbow and the other on the back of your wrist. He or she will then try to push your wrist inward while you try to resist outward. Then do the same test on the affected side. If the rotator cuff on the affected side is weaker or if the test causes pain in the neck or shoulder region, this is a positive sign that the rotator cuff has strained, which indicates a possible strain of the levator scapulae.

MUSCLE TEST POSITION—EXTERNAL ROTATION   **MUSCLE TEST POSITION—INTERNAL ROTATION**

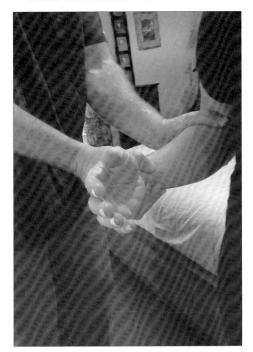
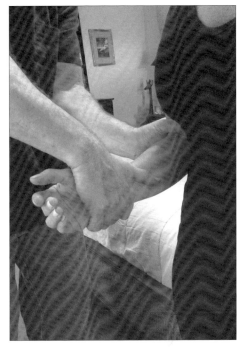

The next test, which is composed of two tests, will help determine which of the shoulder blade stabilizing muscles has been strained. Again you will need someone to provide the resistance for this test. To do the first test, raise both your arms out to the side up to shoulder height and bend your elbows to 90 degrees, keeping your forearms and palms facing down. Have your helper place his or her hands on the tops of your wrists and apply force toward the ground while you try to resist. For the next test, raise both your arms out to the side up to shoulder height, keeping your elbows straight and your forearms and palms facing down. Again have your helper place his or her hands on the tops of your wrists and apply pressure toward the ground while you try to resist.

MUSCLE TEST—SHOULDER FLEXION

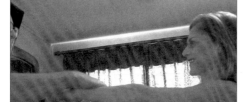

MUSCLE TEST—SHOULDER ABDUCTION

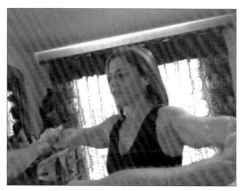

If the muscle testing shows greater weakness or pain elicited with the arms in front of you, then the serratus anterior muscle must be strengthened. If more pain or weakness is elicited with the arms to the side, then the rhomboids and mid-traps must be strengthened.

Flexibility Testing: Looking at the flexibility of the rotator cuff will help determine the extent of the strain to this muscle group along with which exercises should be performed to resolve the strain. To test the flexibility of the rotator cuff, you will again need your helper. Raise your arm on the painful side out to the side up to shoulder height and bend your elbow 90 degrees, keeping your forearm and palm facing down. Your helper will stand at the elbow of your outstretched arm and place one hand at the back of your shoulder and the inside of his or her elbow under your elbow. The goal here is to stabilize your upper arm. With the other hand, he or she will begin to apply pressure to the top of your wrist. You will not resist this. Your helper will continue this pressure, rotating your shoulder while circling your forearm down but keeping your upper arm in place. This test should be performed slowly, and as soon as pain is elicited, the position of the shoulder rotation should be noted.

FLEXIBILITY TEST INTO INTERNAL ROTATION

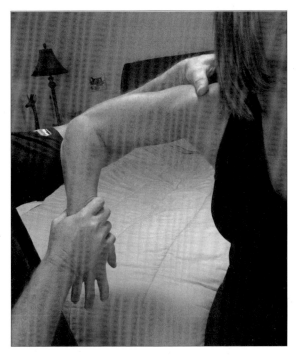

If the rotator cuff can be stretched to 90 degrees of internal rotation (moved so your forearm is perpendicular to the floor) without pain, then you will simply work to strengthen this muscle group. However, if the rotator cuff cannot be stretched to 90 degrees of internal rotation without pain, then you must first work to lengthen this muscle group before strengthening it.

If you have performed all these tests and found positive results, you have confirmation that the cause of your neck pain is a strain of the rotator cuff and shoulder blade stabilizing muscles. The great thing about this is that it is likely that your pain can not only be resolved but also prevented from recurring. Simply perform the following stretching and strengthening exercises:

1. External Rotation (page 234) or Internal Rotation (page 234): If you need to stretch your rotator cuff before strengthening it, perform the Internal Rotation until your rotator cuff can be stretched to 90

degrees without pain. Once you have done this, you can move on to the External Rotation. If you don't need to work on lengthening this muscle, simply do the External Rotation.

2. Protraction Punch (page 238) or Lat Pulldown with Neutral Bar or Elastic Band (page 235): If you need to strengthen your serratus anterior muscle, do the Protraction Punch. If you need to strengthen your rhomboids and mid-traps, do the Lat Pulldown with Neutral Bar or Elastic Band.

3. Posterior Deltoids (page 237)

4. Skull Crushers (page 239)

5. Lower Trap Exercise (page 236)

MIGRAINES AND CLUSTER HEADACHES

While migraines and cluster headaches aren't technically neck pain, they are commonly associated with neck dysfunction, so I'd like to address them here.

Before I talk about the possible muscular causes of headaches, I want to stress the importance of diagnostic tests to verify that the headaches are not the symptom of a serious condition. Cancer, meningitis, allergy reactions, and sinus issues can all create headaches, and CAT scans, blood tests, and any other types of tests should first be used to confirm or refute whether these conditions exist.

But what if all the tests are negative? What if nothing shows up? What happens now? What I've found is that migraine or cluster headaches are often the result of muscle tension coming from the neck as a result of improper alignment of the head.

This improper alignment comes from an imbalance in strength between the muscles in the front of your body and the muscles in the back of the body—pecs (chest muscles), anterior deltoids (front shoulder muscles), and biceps (front upper arm muscles) versus the middle trapezius and rhomboids (the muscles between the shoulder blades), posterior deltoids (back shoulder muscles), and triceps (back upper arm muscles). As a general rule, the muscles in the front of your body are stronger than those in the back of your body because most activities are performed in front of the body—thus the front-of-body muscles are worked more regularly.

As a result of increased strength, these front-of-body muscles also tend to shorten, pulling the head and shoulders forward and creating an improper posture called forward head posture and forward shoulder posture. As the shoulders move forward, the shoulder blades move outward, away from the spine, and any muscles that attach from the skull or spine to the shoulder blades become overstretched. An overstretched muscle loses its ability to create force and perform its functional task.

The muscles that I've found most associated with headaches are the levator scapulae and the upper trapezius, both of which run from the shoulder blade to the upper cervical spine and skull. It is important to understand that the muscles don't attach to the bone itself; rather, they attach to a connective covering that surrounds the bone, called periosteum. The periosteum covers the entire skull.

If the muscles attaching to the periosteum (the levator scapulae and the upper trapezius) are stretched because of muscle imbalance, they pull on the periosteum, thus causing tension on the skull. This leads to headaches at different areas of the head through the mechanism of strained muscles pulling excessively on the skull.

To see if this could be the cause of your headaches—again, only *after* tests that rule out a more severe condition—you will do the tests I've listed above. If your headaches seem to be on both sides, you will perform the tests associated with pain on both sides of the neck. If your headaches seem to be only on one side, do the tests associated with one-sided neck pain. The findings and exercises recommended also apply to headaches.

CHAPTER 6

THE
MID-BACK

MUSCULATURE OF THE UPPER, MID-, AND LOWER BACK

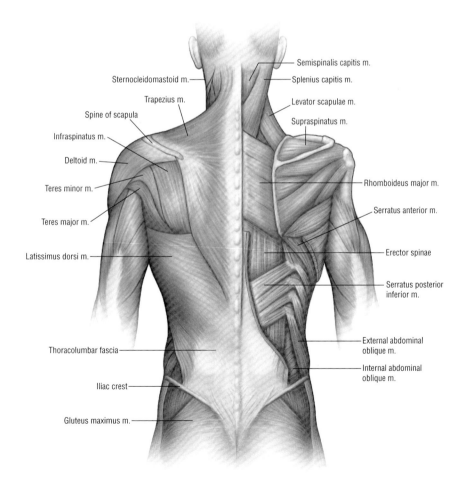

Semispinalis capitis m.

Sternocleidomastoid m.

Splenius capitis m.

Trapezius m.

Levator scapulae m.

Spine of scapula

Supraspinatus m.

Infraspinatus m.

Deltoid m.

Teres minor m.

Rhomboideus major m.

Serratus anterior m.

Teres major m.

Erector spinae

Latissimus dorsi m.

Serratus posterior
inferior m.

External abdominal
oblique m.

Thoracolumbar fascia

Internal abdominal
oblique m.

Iliac crest

Gluteus maximus m.

The mid-back region stems from the bottom of your neck to the top of your lower back, incorporating the area between the shoulder blades. It is typically thought of as the thoracic spine region. In this chapter you will find a description of the muscle groups possibly involved in creating pain in your mid-back, along with clinical tests to confirm which muscle is emitting the pain. Once you have determined where the pain is coming from, please go to the Appendix to learn the muscle-strengthening exercises that will help resolve your pain.

PAIN ON BOTH SIDES OF THE MID-BACK

If you have pain across your mid-back—not simply on one side—you will likely find that you have an imbalance in strength between the muscles in the front of your body and the muscles in the back of the body—pecs (chest muscles), anterior deltoids (front shoulder muscles), and biceps (front upper arm muscles) versus the middle trapezius and rhomboids (the muscles between the shoulder blades), posterior deltoids (back shoulder muscles), and triceps (back upper arm muscles). As a general rule, the muscles in the front of your body are stronger than those in the back of your body because most activities are performed in front of the body—thus the front-of-body muscles are worked more regularly.

If the imbalance between these muscle groups increases significantly enough, the muscles in the back are no longer able to act as a counterforce to the muscles in the front and the shoulders pull forward, creating an improper posture known as forward head and shoulder posture. In this posture, the shoulder blades are pulled outward, away from the spine, and any muscle that attaches to the shoulder blade from the skull or spine becomes overstretched.

If this posture is sustained for a long enough period, it will make the curvature of the thoracic spine even more dramatic, creating an almost C-like shape to the spine, a condition called kyphosis. This causes the rhomboid muscles and the mid-traps muscles that attach from the spine to the shoulder blades to become overstretched. By overstretching, they lose their ability to create force, which causes them to strain. A strained rhomboid or mid-trap can emit pain at their attachment to the spine or anywhere between the spine and the shoulder blade.

To figure out if the rhomboids or mid-traps are strained, you will perform a number of clinical tests, including a posture analysis, palpation, and muscle testing.

Posture Analysis: Let's look at your posture. As I mentioned, people with pain across the whole mid-back often have forward head and shoulder posture. To confirm whether or not you have this posture, have somebody take a full-length photo of you from the side. Simply stand how you would comfortably and normally.

Once you have the photo, look at the position of your ear in relationship to your shoulder. If your ear lines up in front of the shoulder when looking at yourself from the side, that describes forward head posture. To determine if you also have forward shoulder posture, look at your shoulder in respect to your hip, knee, and ankle. These joints should roughly align. If the shoulder is in front of your hip, knee, and ankle, you have forward shoulder posture. If this improper posture is found, you now have a corroborating finding that your mid-back pain is the result of the muscle imbalance described.

Palpation: Now let's do some palpation, or the touching of tissues. Remember, the goal of this test is to elicit pain in order to identify which muscle is causing your mid-back pain.

With most people who experience pain across the entire mid-back, pressing on the rhomboid or mid-trap, which run between the spine and the shoulder blade, will increase pain. If this is true for you, you now have yet another corroborating finding that the cause of your pain is the muscle imbalance described. Remember, if the pain were coming from a structural variation, such as scoliosis, pain would only be increased by putting pressure on the spine itself. This would be referred pain. If pain is point-tender, coming from the muscle itself, this is not structural.

Muscle Testing: Finally, muscle testing can be performed to see if there is a muscle imbalance between the chest muscles and muscles between the shoulder blades. This test requires help from someone else. Simply raise your arm out to the side up to shoulder height and bend your elbow to 90 degrees, keeping your forearm and hand parallel to the ground. Your helper will be testing how forcefully you are able to resist him or her—both while you are pushing backward and while you are pushing forward. First, you will test your forward strength by having your helper place one hand on the back of your shoulder and the other inside the bend of your elbow. Press your arm forward as powerfully as you can while your helper resists. Next, have him or her put one hand on the front of your shoulder and one on the back of your elbow. Press your arm backward as powerfully as you can while your helper resists. If it is much harder to resist the forward press than the backward press, you have confirmed that a muscle imbalance exists between the pecs and muscles between the shoulder blades. It is not necessary to perform the test on both sides. If the imbalance is found on one side, you can conclude that the same would be found on the other side.

MUSCLE TESTING—ANTERIOR TORSO MUSCLES　　　**MUSCLE TESTING—POSTERIOR TORSO MUSCLES**

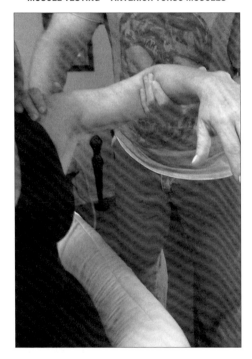
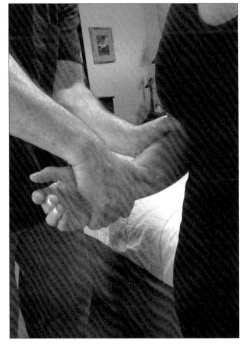

If you have forward shoulder posture and/or kyphosis (excessive hunching of the mid-back), you will likely find that your pecs are much stronger than the muscles between your shoulder blades.

If you have performed all these tests and found positive results, you have confirmation that the cause of your mid-back pain is a muscle imbalance. The great thing about this is that it is likely that your pain can not only be resolved but also prevented from recurring. Simply perform the following strengthening exercises:

1. Posterior Deltoids (page 237)

2. Lat Pulldown with Neutral Bar or Elastic Band (page 235)

3. Skull Crushers (page 239)

4. Lower Trap Exercise (page 236)

SINGLE-SIDED MID-BACK PAIN

If you have pain on only one side of your mid-back, a problem with your shoulder and/or shoulder blade is a likely cause.

The shoulder joint is composed of the upper arm bone and the end of the shoulder blade. When the shoulder joint is moved, the shoulder blade glides on the rib cage. There are a few muscles that are responsible for this—some of the muscles help move it, while others work to keep it pressed tight to the rib cage to allow for the gliding motion. For the shoulder blade to move correctly, these muscles—the stabilizing muscles and the moving muscles—must work together.

Remember that the mid-traps and rhomboids (responsible for stabilizing the shoulder blade) and the rotator cuff (responsible for stabilizing the shoulder joint) are intimately connected. The strain of one can easily cause a strain of the other. In the case of shoulder function causing mid-back pain, this is typically due to a rotator cuff strain (not a tear). Not only is the rotator cuff one of the key muscle groups involved in maintaining proper mechanics of the shoulder joint, it is also responsible for keeping the upper portion of the upper arm bone in the shoulder joint.

A strain of the rhomboids or mid-traps leads to an instability of the shoulder blade against the rib cage. In turn, the rotator cuff has to work harder to keep the upper arm bone in the shoulder joint. The excess load caused by the lack of stability is enough to cause the rotator cuff to strain, which in turn can cause the rhomboids or mid-traps to strain to the point of emitting pain.

If you experience pain between your shoulder blades or along the part of your spine that is in line with the shoulder blades, this means that the mid-traps and rhomboids have strained. If the pain is just a bit lower—along the portion of your spine just below your shoulder blades yet above the top of your lumbar spine—this means that the lower trap muscle has strained.

The lower trap's role in shoulder function is very important. It not only stabilizes the shoulder blade along with the mid-trap/rhomboids, the levator scapulae, and the serratus anterior, but also pulls it down the rib cage during the upper end of shoulder motion. If you raise your arm higher than shoulder height, the thrust of this motion is achieved through the shoulder blade being pulled down the back by the lower trap muscle. The lower trap is a fairly long muscle that starts at the shoulder blade and runs down to the lower thoracic spine.

To confirm the cause of the pain at either the upper or lower thoracic spine region, you will need to do some palpation, muscle testing, and flexibility testing.

Palpation: First, let's do some palpation, or the touching of tissues. Remember, the goal of this test is to elicit pain in order to identify which muscle is causing your mid-back pain. Lie on your stomach and have someone palpate the whole of your mid-back—from the upper section between the shoulder blades down to the bottom of the rib cage. If you are able to bring forth a pain signal in either the mid-traps and rhomboids or the lower traps, you will have your first clue as to which muscle needs to be strengthened.

Muscle Testing: Muscle testing of the rotator cuff will help confirm that the mid-trap/rhomboids or the lower trap muscle has strained. You will muscle test the rotator cuff to check for a mid-trap/rhomboid strain, and you will test the lower trap itself for strain.

To muscle test the rotator cuff, you will need someone to help you. On the unaffected side, keeping the top of your arm flush against your body, bend your elbow to 90 degrees. Your forearm will be facing your body and your hand will be thumb side up, as if you're positioning it to shake hands with someone. Next, have your helper place one hand on the outside of your elbow and the other on the back of the wrist. He or she will then try to push your wrist inward while you try to resist outward. Then do the same test on the affected side. If the rotator cuff on the affected side is weaker or if the test causes pain in the mid-back or shoulder region, this is a positive sign that the rotator cuff has strained, which indicates a possible strain of the mid-traps/rhomboids.

MUSCLE TESTING—SHOULDER EXTERNAL ROTATION

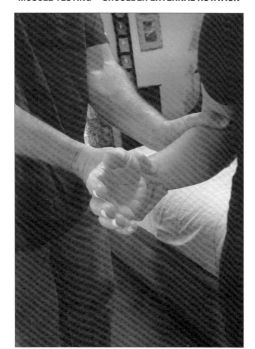

MUSCLE TESTING—SHOULDER INTERNAL ROTATION

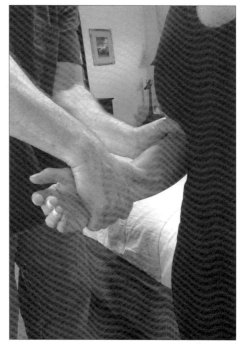

The next test, which is composed of two tests, will help determine which of the shoulder blade stabilizing muscles has been strained. Again you will need someone to provide the resistance for this test. To do the first test, raise both your arms in front of you to shoulder height with the elbows straight, keeping your forearms and palms facing down. Have your helper place his or her hands on the tops of your wrists and apply force toward the ground while you try to resist. For the next test, raise both your arms out to the side up to shoulder height, keeping your elbows straight and your forearms and palms facing down. Again have your helper place his or her hands on the tops of your wrists and apply pressure toward the ground while you try to resist.

MUSCLE TESTING—SHOULDER FLEXION

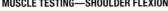

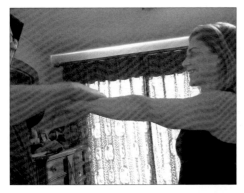

MUSCLE TESTING—SHOULDER ABDUCTION

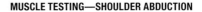

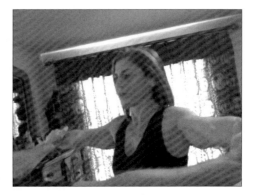

If the muscle testing shows greater weakness or pain elicited with the arms in front of you, then the serratus anterior muscle must be strengthened. If more pain or weakness is elicited with the arms to the side, then the rhomboids and mid-traps must be strengthened.

To test for a lower trap strain, you will again need someone to help you. Place your arms halfway between in front of you and to your side with the elbows straight and the shoulders at about a 140-degree angle with the hands facing inward toward one another. Your helper will then put pressure on the tops of your wrists, trying to push down while you resist. If it is easier to push the arm down on the side with the mid-back region pain, this is another indicator that the pain is caused by a lower trap muscle strain.

MUSCLE TESTING—LOWER TRAPEZIUS

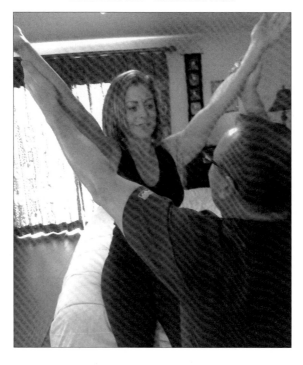

Flexibility Testing: Looking at the flexibility of the rotator cuff will help determine the extent of the strain to this muscle group along with which exercises should be performed to resolve the strain. To test the flexibility of the rotator cuff, you will again need your helper. Raise your arm on the painful side out to the side up to shoulder height and bend your elbow 90 degrees, keeping your forearm and palm facing down. Your helper will stand at the elbow of your outstretched arm and place one hand at the back of your shoulder and the inside of his or her elbow under your elbow. The goal here is to stabilize your upper arm. With the other hand, he or she will begin to apply pressure to the top of your wrist. You will not resist this. Your helper will continue this pressure, rotating your shoulder while circling your forearm down but keeping your upper arm in place. This test should be performed slowly, and as soon as pain is elicited, the position of the shoulder rotation should be noted.

MUSCLE TESTING—SHOULDER INTERNAL ROTATION

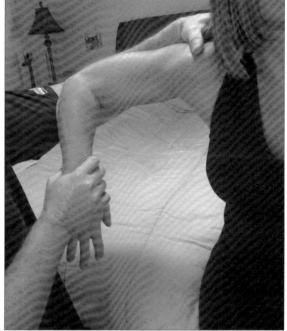

If the rotator cuff can be stretched to 90 degrees of internal rotation (moved so your forearm is perpendicular to the floor) without pain, then you will simply work to strengthen this muscle group. However, if the rotator cuff cannot be stretched to 90 degrees of internal rotation without pain, then you must first work to lengthen this muscle group before strengthening it.

No matter if you found a strain of the rotator cuff, mid-traps/rhomboids, or lower traps, you will work to strengthen all of these. The reason I asked you to determine whether the strain was coming from the mid-traps/rhomboids or the lower traps is because these muscle groups are in distinct locations, and if your pain is in a specific location, it is important to understand which tissue is emitting the pain signal. Also, many people are often helped by incorporating massage intermittently into their treatment. This massage would focus on the strained muscles. To strengthen and stretch the muscles associated with mid-back pain on one side, please do the following exercises:

1. External Rotation (page 234) or Internal Rotation (page 234): If you need to stretch your rotator cuff before strengthening it, perform the Internal Rotation until your rotator cuff can be stretched to 90 degrees without pain. Once you have done this, you can move on to the External Rotation. If you don't need to work on lengthening this muscle, simply do the External Rotation.

2. Protraction Punch (page 238) or Lat Pulldown with Neutral Bar or Elastic Band (page 235): If you need to strengthen your serratus anterior muscle, do the Protraction Punch. If you need to strengthen your rhomboids and mid-traps, do the Lat Pulldown with Neutral Bar or Elastic Band.

3. Posterior Deltoids (page 237)

4. Skull Crushers (page 239)

5. Lower Trap Exercise (page 236)

CHAPTER 7

THE
LOWER
BACK

LOWER BACK MUSCULATURE

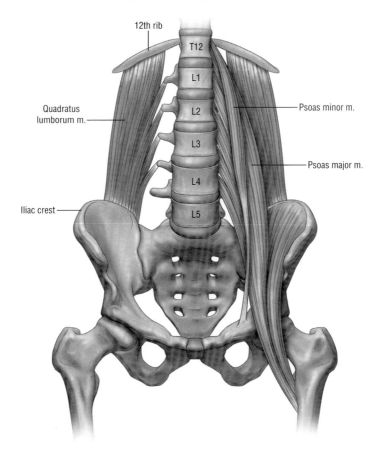

12th rib

T12

L1

Quadratus
lumborum m.

L2

Psoas minor m.

L3

Psoas major m.

L4

Iliac crest

L5

QUADRATUS LUMBORUM

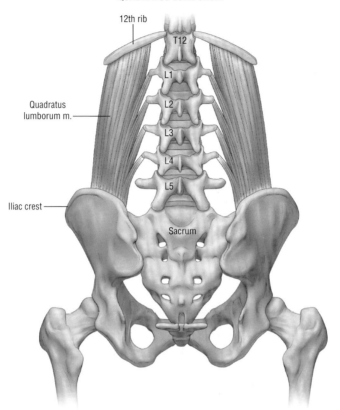

Lower back pain is one of the most common types of chronic pain around. One reason for this is because the lower back is the transition point between the upper and lower body, which makes it very susceptible to strain and injury. Why? Because any time an activity is performed with the arms or the legs, the lower back comes into play. It supports the torso so the muscles that attach from the torso to the arm or leg can move the limb. The lower back is also involved in any weight-bearing activity. Even when you are sitting, if your back is not supported, the lower back is being challenged.

Another important thing to understand about the lower back region is that the pelvis, which makes up the bottom portion of this region, is constantly changing position. Most other joints are pretty much stable in their position; one bone simply moves on the other bone at the joint. In the lower back region, the rib cage and pelvis are constantly changing in relationship to each other. This creates the possibility of severe changes in muscle length occurring that strain the muscles of the lower back.

The final reason that this area is one of the most commonly complained about is actually a misunderstanding of what this area is. The lower back and the gluteal region are in close proximity to each other, and, often, the medical establishment treats them as one area. However, they are distinctly different. So before you jump into the work of this chapter, please verify that your pain is indeed in your lower back and not in your gluteal region. The delineating line between the lower back and the gluteal region is the pelvic rim. Most people perceive this as their hips. Put your hands on your hips with your thumbs in the back. Now imagine a line running across the back of your body from thumb to thumb. This is the separating line between the lower back and the gluteal region. If your pain is below this line, it is in the gluteal region, so please head to the next chapter. If your pain is above the line, it is in the lower back, so stick around here.

In this chapter you will find a description of the muscle groups possibly involved in creating pain in your lower back, along with clinical tests to confirm which muscle is emitting the pain. There are various options for each type of pain, so before you start any of the exercises in the program, make sure to read through and do the tests for each possibility. This will ensure that you have properly identified which muscle is emitting pain, and thus you will be sure you are doing the proper exercises to correct it.

PAIN ON BOTH SIDES OF THE BACK

Possibility 1: Muscle Imbalance Between Quads and Hip Flexors Versus Glutes and Hamstrings

By far the most common reason for pain across the lower back is a muscle imbalance that develops between the quads and hip flexors (the muscles on the front of the body) versus the glutes and hamstrings (the muscles on the back of the body). This is a common scenario because most functional activities—whether it's climbing stairs, sitting down, or getting up—are performed in front of us. This causes the quads and hip flexors to be used more often and thus become stronger than the glutes and hamstrings. If this imbalance increases enough, the quads and hip flexors will shorten. Because the quads attach to the front of the pelvis, their shortening will pull the front of the pelvis down, causing the back of the pelvis to rise. The rise of the back of the pelvis causes an excessive arching of the lower back, which, in turn, causes the lower back muscles to shorten. Once shortened, the lower back muscles lose their ability to create force and perform their task of supporting the torso. This causes these muscles to strain and emit pain across the lower back.

To verify that this is the cause of your lower back pain, you'll do the following clinical tests: posture analysis, flexibility testing, muscle testing, and palpation.

Posture Analysis: The first indicator of a muscle imbalance between the quads and hamstrings is an abnormal positioning of the pelvis. There are two bony points that can be felt on the pelvic bone: the anterior superior iliac spine (ASIS) on the front of the pelvis and the posterior superior iliac spine (PSIS) on the back of the pelvis.

ANATOMY OF THE PELVIS

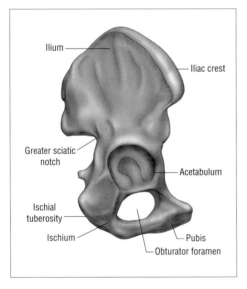

ANTERIOR AND NEUTRAL POSTURE

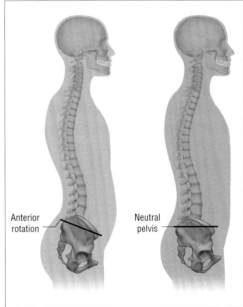

NEUTRAL PELVIC POSTURE

ANTERIOR TILT PELVIC POSTURE

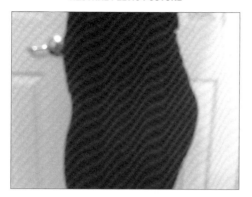
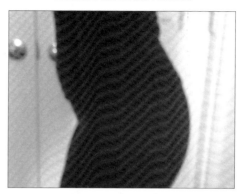

When there is a muscle imbalance resulting from the quads being stronger than the hamstrings, the ASIS will be drawn down and will be much lower than the PSIS. To judge the alignment of your ASIS and PSIS, simply look at yourself from the side in the mirror, standing as you would normally stand. Feel for these two landmarks on your pelvis, and draw a line between the ASIS and PSIS. If the line angles up from front to back, this is a sign that you may have this imbalance. If this is the case, you will also notice an excessive arch or curve in your lower back.

Flexibility Testing: Next, let's look at flexibility of the quads and hamstrings. If the quads are found to be very tight and the hamstrings are found to be excessively flexible, this is another indicator that the quads are stronger than the hamstrings.

To test the quads' flexibility, stand holding on to a sturdy object with one hand and then grab the ankle of the leg on the other side. Try to pull your ankle to your buttocks. If you can't reach your heel to your buttocks while also keeping your knee slightly behind the hip, then your quads are tight.

FLEXIBILITY TESTING—QUADS

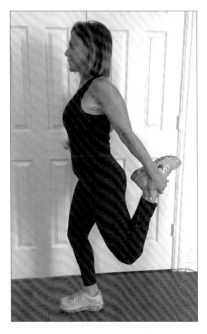

Now test your hamstrings. Lie on your back with one knee bent and the foot of that leg on the surface where you're lying. Have somebody try to raise your other leg with the knee straight. You should be able to raise your leg so it is pointing straight up. This is considered normal range of motion of the hamstrings. If you can go farther than straight up, then you are hyperflexible with respect to the hamstrings.

FLEXIBILITY TESTING—HAMSTRINGS

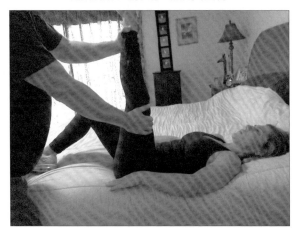

A tight quad with either a normal or hyperflexible hamstring is an indication of a muscle imbalance between the quads and the hamstrings.

Muscle Testing: Now let's look at muscle testing. To test the quads and hamstrings for muscle strength, sit on a sturdy chair. You will need somebody to help you test your strength. You will be sitting with one foot on the floor and one foot off the floor with the knee bent to about 70 degrees. Your helper will place one hand on the top of the thigh and one in front of the ankle. You will try to extend (straighten) the knee while your helper tries to stop you at the ankle. This is the test for quad strength. Now have your helper take his or her hand and put it behind the ankle. From the same start position as before (the knee bent to 70 degrees), try to bend your knee more while your helper tries to stop you. This is how you test the strength of the hamstrings. If the kicking out is much stronger than the pulling backward, this is another indicator of the muscle imbalance causing the pain at the lower back.

MUSCLE TESTING—QUADS

MUSCLE TESTING—HAMSTRINGS

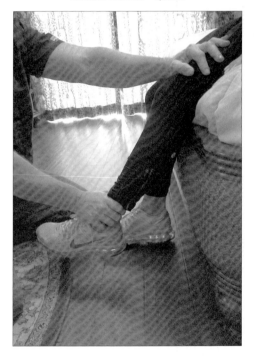
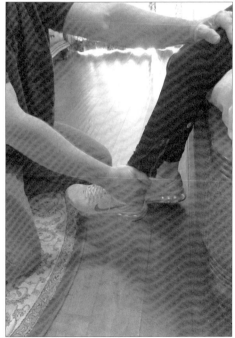

Palpation: Finally, we can palpate, or touch, the lower back region to see if we can determine which tissue is emitting the pain signal. Look at the diagram at the beginning of this chapter that shows the quadratus lumborum. These are the main muscles that span the lower back region. Press along the whole muscle, from the attachment to the rib cage to the attachment to the pelvis. Pain from the strained muscles may be exhibited at any location along the muscle. If the pain you are experiencing is increased by pressing on these muscles, this is final confirmation that the cause of the lower back pain is from strained lower back muscles, which resulted from a muscle imbalance between the quads and hamstrings.

If you have determined that this is definitively the cause of your pain, the key to resolving it is to stretch the quads and strengthen the glutes, hamstrings, and hip abductors. The exercises to be performed are:

1. Quad Stretch (page 249)
2. Hamstring Curl (page 240)
3. Straight Leg Deadlifts (page 246)
4. Hip Extension (page 242)
5. Hip Abduction (page 241)

Possibility 2: Forward Center of Mass

In the case of a muscle imbalance between the quads and hamstrings causing the pain across the lower back, an increased arching of the lower back was the only postural deficit found. In this instance, your ear and shoulder are still centered over your hip joint. However, if your ear and shoulder are in front of the hip joint, your pain may be coming from something referred to as forward center of mass. This postural variation makes you look as if you are bent forward from the hip joint.

POSTURAL ANALYSIS—NORMAL POSTURE   **POSTURAL ANALYSIS—FORWARD CENTER OF MASS**

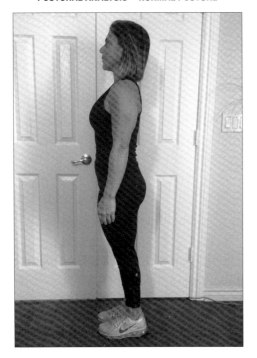 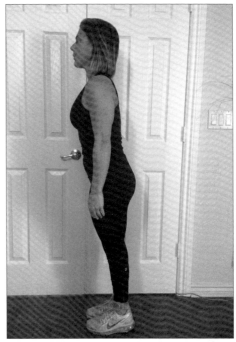

This posture is associated with an imbalance between the hip flexors (iliopsoas) and glutes. The hip flexors attach from the lumbar spine to the hip joint, and if they shorten excessively, they pull the lumbar spine forward. This not only causes an excessive arching of the lower back but draws the torso forward at the hip, creating a forward center of mass position in which the person feels they are weight bearing more through the balls of the feet than the heels. The shortened hip flexors also make it difficult to stand upright. Another classic indicator of this imbalance is difficulty standing up after sitting for a while. When you're sitting, your hip flexors are shortened, and they have difficulty lengthening upon standing up.

With the hip flexors shortened, they can strain and emit pain at their attachment to the lumbar spine. And if the hip flexors spasm, the pain can be so intense at the spine that it could lead to an inability to move from a hip-flexed position. The big difference between the pain we discussed in the previous section and the pain associated with forward center of mass is the location of the pain. The forward center of mass caused by the strained and shortened hip flexors will cause pain close to the spine rather than along the width of the lower back. This pain close to the spine can easily convince someone that the pain is coming from a structural element of the spine, but this isn't necessarily the case.

To determine if the forward center of mass position is what's causing your lower back pain, you'll analyze your posture, and then do some flexibility testing and palpation.

Posture Analysis: The most obvious clinical indicator of a forward center of mass being the cause of the lower back pain is the difficulty or inability of the person to stand upright. Look at the side view of yourself in the mirror again, standing as you would normally stand. Notice where your ear and shoulder are in relation to your hip. If they are in front of the hip, this is an indication that there is an imbalance between your hip flexors and glutes. You will also notice that you are bearing weight more through the balls of the feet than your heels.

Flexibility Testing: The next indicator to look at is the flexibility of the hip flexors. To test this, lie on a surface where one leg can hang off, such as a table. Lie on your back with both knees bent and your feet on the surface. Next, grab and pull one knee into your chest. Then try to hang the other leg off the surface. If your hanging leg cannot reach down to the point where the thigh is in line with the torso (parallel to the ground) and the lower leg is pointing toward the ground, then you have a tight hip flexor. For some people, the hip flexors may be so shortened that even attempting to get into this position is too painful.

FLEXIBILITY TESTING—HIP FLEXORS

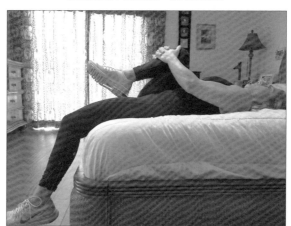

Another aspect of flexibility that indicates a forward center of mass is tight quads *and* hamstrings. Typically, one or the other of these muscles will be tight, indicating a muscle imbalance. However, in the case of an imbalance between the hip flexors and glutes, both are tight. The quads are tight because of the muscle imbalance between the quads and hamstrings. The hamstrings have tightened because they are overworking. With a forward center of mass posture, the hip-flexed position creates a load that is in front of the heel. This load must be supported by muscles in the back of the legs. The hamstrings constantly overworking to support this excess load strains and shortens them. This creates the unique situation where both your quads and hamstrings are shortened.

To test the quads' flexibility, stand holding on to a sturdy object with one hand and then grab the ankle of the leg on the other side. Try to pull your ankle to your buttocks. If you can't reach your heel to your buttocks while also keeping your knee slightly behind the hip, then your quads are tight.

Now test your hamstrings. Lie on your back with one knee bent and the foot of that leg on the floor. Have somebody try to raise your other leg with the knee straight. You should be able to raise your leg so it is pointing straight up. This is considered normal range of motion of the hamstrings. If you cannot do this, you have a tight hamstring.

A tight quad with a tight hamstring is an indication of a muscle imbalance between the hip flexors and the glutes and a forward center of mass as the cause of the lower back pain.

Palpation: Next, you can palpate the hip flexors to see if the pain is elicited from pressing on the muscle itself. To feel for the hip flexors, lie on your back on a comfortable but firm surface. Feel for the anterior superior iliac spine (ASIS). Once you identify this landmark, move your fingers toward the belly button about one to two inches and then move your fingers down toward the feet about one or two inches. You should be able to feel a thickened, almost ball-like tissue. This is the hip flexors. Press on this tissue and see if pain is elicited. If pain is experienced, this is another indicator that the pain at the lower back is caused by a forward center of mass.

The location of your lower back pain is the final clinical indicator to determine if forward center of mass is the cause. Although the pain will be felt on both sides of the lower back, in this case the pain will be experienced closer to the spine.

If the cause of your pain was found to be an imbalance between the hip flexors and glutes, or a forward center of mass, the key to resolving your pain is to stretch the hip flexors and quads and strengthen the glutes, hamstrings, and hip abductors. The exercises to be performed are:

1. Quad Stretch (page 249)
2. Hip Flexor Stretch (page 248)
3. Hamstring Curl (page 240)
4. Straight Leg Deadlifts (page 246)
5. Hip Extension (page 242)
6. Hip Abduction (page 241)

Possibility 3: Strained Quads Causing Shortened Hamstrings

The final possibility for lower back pain on both sides of the back is strained quads that shorten your hamstrings and create a flattening of your back. This is actually somewhat rare, accounting for only about 10 percent of cases. Generally I see this in people who have had knee injuries or who have been bedridden for a period of time. There is typically a reason why the quads haven't been working normally and have weakened to the point where the hamstrings could overtake them in strength.

In this case, the shortened hamstrings are pulling the back of the pelvis down, creating a posterior tilt—the back lower than the front. This creates an increase in space between the bottom of the rib cage and the top of the pelvis in which the normal arch of the lower back is replaced with a flattened lower back. Since the lower back muscles attach from the bottom of the rib cage and top of the pelvis, they become overstretched and lose their ability to create force to support the torso. This causes them to strain and emit pain across the lower back.

POSTERIOR TILT

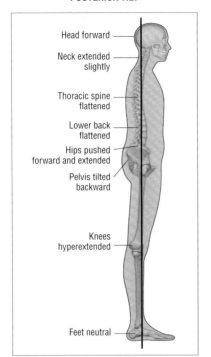

- Head forward
- Neck extended slightly
- Thoracic spine flattened
- Lower back flattened
- Hips pushed forward and extended
- Pelvis tilted backward
- Knees hyperextended
- Feet neutral

POSTERIOR TILT

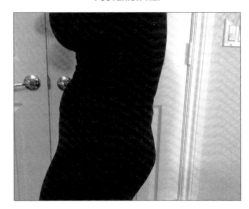

To determine if strained quads and shortened hamstrings are the cause of your lower back pain, you will analyze your posture, and then do flexibility testing, muscle testing, and palpation.

Posture Analysis: The first indicator to look at is posture. You will again look at a side view of yourself in the mirror, standing as you would normally stand. Then identify the ASIS and the PSIS. If the ASIS is higher than the PSIS, this is an indication that you have shortened hamstrings. You will also notice that your lower back looks flattened with no arch present.

ANATOMY OF PELVIS

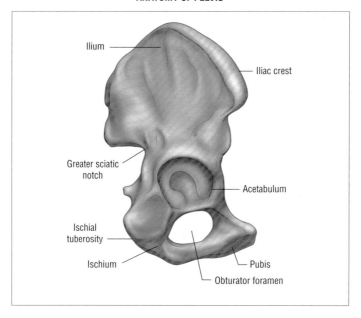

POSTERIOR AND ANTERIOR TILT OF PELVIS

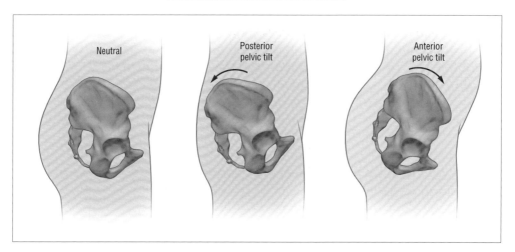

Flexibility Testing: Next, you can look at flexibility. To test the quads' flexibility, stand holding on to a sturdy object with one hand and then grab the ankle of the leg on the other side. Try to pull your ankle to your buttocks. If you can't reach your heel to your buttocks while also keeping your knee slightly behind the hip, then your quads are tight.

Now test your hamstrings. Lie on your back with one knee bent and the foot of that leg on the floor. Have somebody try to raise your other leg with the knee straight. You should be able to raise your leg so it is pointing straight up. This is considered normal range of motion of the hamstrings. If you cannot do this, you have a tight hamstring.

If the quads are found to be normal length, but the hamstrings are found to be shortened, this is an indication of the shortened hamstrings pulling on the lower back excessively, causing the lower back pain.

Muscle Testing: Next, you can muscle test the quads and hamstrings. To do this, sit on a sturdy chair. You will need somebody to help you test your strength. You will be sitting with one foot on the floor and one foot off the floor with the knee bent to about 70 degrees. Your helper will place one hand on the top of the thigh and one in front of the ankle. You will try to extend (straighten) the knee while your helper tries to stop you at the ankle. This is the test for quad strength. Now have your helper take his or her hand and put it behind the ankle. From the same start position as before (the knee bent to 70 degrees), try to bend your knee more while your helper tries to stop you. This is how you test the strength of the hamstrings. If the pulling backward is stronger than the kicking out, this is another indication that the shortened hamstrings are causing the lower back pain.

Palpation: Finally, palpate the lower back and feel for the lower back muscles, the quadratus lumborum (QLs), the main muscles that span the lower back region. Press along the whole muscle, from the attachment to the rib cage to the attachment to the pelvis. Pain anywhere along this muscle will confirm that the tissue emitting the pain signal is the lower back muscle.

If you have confirmed that an imbalance in which your hamstrings are stronger than your quads is the cause of your lower back pain, then you will want to do the following stretching and strengthening exercises:

1. Hamstring Stretch (page 248)
2. Knee Extension (page 242)
3. Squats (page 245)
4. Hip Abduction (page 241)

SINGLE-SIDED BACK PAIN

Possibility 1: Strained Gluteus Medius (Glute Med) Causing Lower Muscle to Overwork

If you have pain on just one side of your lower back, the most likely cause is a strained hip muscle called the gluteus medius (glute med). This strain can be either on the same side as the pain or on the opposite side.

The gluteus medius plays a pivotal role in supporting you, especially when standing on one leg, as in the case of walking. The glute med keeps the pelvis level when standing on one leg so balance is maintained. If the glute med is weak, the pelvis on the side opposite of which you are standing will begin to drop toward the floor. This shifts your center of mass from over the leg you are standing on to the midline of the body. If this happens, you will want to put your opposite foot on the floor quickly to prevent yourself from falling.

The glute med can strain for a number of reasons, including compensating for the weakness of the other muscles involved in weight-bearing activities. Ultimately, with the glute med straining, support of the pelvis is compromised. Since the lower back muscles are responsible for support of the torso and they work so strongly in conjunction with the glute meds, straining of the glute meds will cause the lower back muscles to overwork and strain as well, emitting pain at the lower back.

The lower back muscles can strain either on the same side as the strained glute med or on the opposite side. If it is on the same side, it is because the torso stabilizer on the same side as the pelvic stabilizer tried to compensate. If it is on the opposite side, it is because the lower back muscle on the opposite side tried to lift up the pelvis, which was dropping because of the strained glute med. In either case, the relationship between the glute med and the lower back muscles is the cause of the pain at the lower back on one side.

To determine if this is the cause of your one-sided lower back pain—and which glute med is strained (same side as pain or alternate side)—you will do muscle testing, palpation, posture analysis, and a single leg standing test.

Muscle Testing: The first step to confirming a diagnosis of a strained glute med is to test the strength of your glute meds. To perform this test, you'll need the help of someone else. First, lie down on a firm surface on your side. Raise your top leg a few inches, so it runs parallel to the ground. Make sure to keep it in line with your torso, not drifting forward or backward. Have your helper place one hand on your pelvis just above the hip joint and the other on your ankle. Try to push up at the ankle while the person tries to stop you. Then turn over and try the same test with the other leg. If the glute med is weaker on the same side where you are having the lower back pain, this is the first indication that the strained glute med is on the same side as your pain. If the glute med on the opposite side of your body is weaker, this is an indication of strain on the opposite side.

Palpation: Next, you'll palpate the lower back muscles and the glute med. Remember the goal here is to elicit pain in order to identify which muscle is causing your pain. To do this test, you will need someone to help you.

First, lie on your stomach and have your helper feel the lower back region on the side you are having pain. Feel for the lower back muscles, the quadratus lumborum. Have your helper press down on this muscle along its whole length, from the point where it attaches to the rib cage to where it attaches to the pelvis. If pain is felt anywhere along this muscle, you have confirmed that the lower back muscle is the tissue emitting the pain signal.

Next, you'll want to test your glute med. Have your helper find the top of your pelvis, or pelvic rim. Then find the hip joint. The glute med runs along the pelvis and attaches at the hip joint. Your helper will press down in a straight line on the muscle along its entire length, from the top of the pelvis to the hip joint. If pain is experienced during this palpation, then this is another confirming indicator that the glute med on the same side is strained. If you don't experience pain, this is an indication that the strained glute med may be on your opposite side, so you'll also want to palpate the other side. If pressing on that glute med elicits pain, this indicates that you have a strained glute med on the opposite side of your lower back pain.

Posture Analysis: The next thing you'll want to do is look at your posture. Stand in front of a mirror that can provide a full view of you from the front. Place your hands on the rim of your pelvis (most people consider this their hips) and see if one hand is higher than the other. If the lower back muscle has strained because the glute med on the opposite side has strained, it will shorten and pull its attachment to the pelvis higher. This will create the appearance of an elevated pelvis/hip on the side of the lower back pain. So, if the hand on the hip is higher on the side where you are experiencing pain, this indicates that the glute med on the opposite side may be causing your pain. If your hands appear even or higher on the side opposite your lower back pain, this points to a strained glute med on the side where you are experiencing back pain.

STANDING POSTURE—HIPS LEVEL

STANDING POSTURE—HIP HIKED

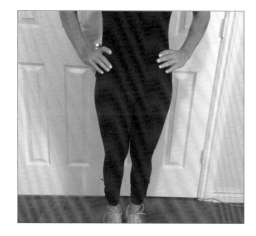 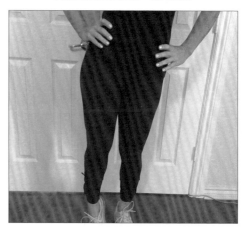

Single Leg Standing Test: The final test to help you confirm which glute med is causing your pain is the single leg standing test. Try to stand on one leg and then try to stand on the opposite leg. If you find it more difficult to stand on one leg or the other, it is likely that the strained glute med is on this side.

If the cause of your pain is found to be a strained glute med, then the key to resolving your pain is to strengthen the glute meds, glutes, and hamstrings on both sides of your body. The exercises to be performed are:

1. Straight Leg Deadlifts (page 246)
2. Hip Abduction (page 241): At first, do these only on the side with the strained glute med. Once it is stronger, move to doing it on both sides.
3. Hamstring Curl (page 240)
4. Hip Extension (page 242)

Possibility 2: Strained Hamstring Causing Quad to Shorten

Another possible cause of lower back pain only on one side is a strained hamstring causing the quad to shorten. The quad is attached to the front of the pelvis, while the hamstring is attached to the back. If the hamstring strains, the imbalance between the quads and hamstrings increases, causing the quads to shorten more, pulling the pelvis down in the front and causing an increased arching at the lower back. The alteration of the pelvis can alter the distance between the bottom of the ribs and the top of the pelvis. Since the lower back muscles attach from the bottom of the rib cage to the top of the pelvis, their length is integrally associated with the distance between these two landmarks. This in turn causes the lower back muscles to shorten, strain, and emit pain at one side of the lower back.

One of the key functional responsibilities of the hamstrings is to slow the lower leg as it swings forward, as with walking or running. The quads cause the swinging, and the hamstrings control it so you are able to place your foot in front of you to start the next step. In this motion, the hamstring is trying to create force while lengthening—a very difficult task, which makes the hamstring very susceptible to strain.

Because muscles all work together in systems, in the case of a strained hamstring, you may experience pain at the back of your thigh and the lower back. Or you may experience pain at the knee and the lower back. Or you may just experience pain at the lower back. It all depends on the extent of the strain of the hamstrings and how much the other muscles have been affected. In any of these cases, the strain of the hamstring must be remedied to resolve the lower back pain.

To see if your one-sided lower back pain is coming from a strained quad, you will do a flexibility test, a muscle test, a posture analysis, and some palpation.

Flexibility Test: The first indicator of this cause would be to look at flexibility of the quad and hamstring on the side where you are experiencing lower back pain.

To test the quad's flexibility, stand holding on to a sturdy object with one hand and then grab the ankle of the leg on the side you are experiencing pain. Try to pull your ankle to your buttocks. If you can't reach your heel to your buttocks while also keeping your knee slightly behind the hip, then your quad is tight.

Now test your hamstring. Lie on your back, bending the knee on the side where you're not experiencing pain and keeping the foot of that leg on the floor. Have somebody try to raise your other leg—the leg on the side where you're experiencing pain—with the knee straight. You should be able to raise your leg so it is pointing straight up. This is considered normal range of motion of the hamstring. If you cannot do this, you have a tight hamstring.

If the quads are tight but the hamstrings are not, this is an indication that a strained hamstring may be causing your single-sided lower back pain.

Muscle Testing: Next, we can look at muscle strength of the quad and hamstring on the side where you are experiencing pain.

To do this, sit on a sturdy chair. You will need somebody to help you test your strength. You will do the testing on the side experiencing the pain while keeping the other foot on the floor. While sitting, lift the foot on the painful side off the floor with the knee bent to about 70 degrees. Your helper will place one hand on the top of the thigh and one in front of the ankle. You will try to extend the knee while the person tries to stop you at the ankle. This is the test for quad strength. Now have the person take his or her hand and put it behind the ankle. From the same start position as before (the knee bent to 70 degrees), try to bend your knee more while the person tries to stop you. This is how you test the strength of the hamstrings. If the pulling backward is weaker than the kicking out, this is another indication that the strained hamstring is causing the lower back pain. You may also find that pain is elicited either at the back of the thigh or at the knee because of the hamstring strain. This would corroborate this diagnosis even more.

Posture Analysis: Next, we can look at posture. Looking at yourself from the side in a mirror, note the position of your pelvis. To do this, you will identify the ASIS and the PSIS (see page 126 if you need more information on this) and look to see if they are even. Do this on one side and then the other. If you find that the ASIS is lower than the PSIS on the side with lower back pain, and either even or less dramatic on the unaffected side, this indicates that the quad is pulling the pelvis forward. You will also notice a greater arching of the lower back on the painful side.

Palpation: Finally, we can look to palpation. Feel along the hamstring muscles and the associated tendons that attach to the knee. See if you can find knots or locations of pain along the muscle and tendons. Compare how the hamstrings feel on the side with lower back pain with how the hamstrings feel on the unaffected side.

You'll also want to palpate your lower back; you'll need someone to help you with this. First, lie on your stomach and have your helper feel the lower back region on the side you are having pain. Feel for the lower back muscles, the quadratus lumborum. Have your helper press down on this muscle along its whole length, from the point where it attaches to the rib cage to where it attaches to the pelvis.

Finding the knotting in the hamstring muscle and knotting and pain elicited in the lower back muscles reinforces the diagnosis that your one-sided lower back pain is due to a strained hamstring.

If the cause of your pain was found to be strained hamstrings and shortened quads, the key to resolving the pain is to stretch the quads and strengthen the hamstrings, glutes, hip abductors, and calf on the side of the body where the pain is being experienced. The exercises to be performed are:

1. Quad Stretch (page 249)
2. Hamstring Curl (page 240)*
3. Straight Leg Deadlifts (page 246)
4. Hip Extension (page 242)
5. Hip Abduction (page 241)
6. Standing Calf Raises (page 246)

* If the hamstrings are found to be shortened (your leg cannot reach to pointing straight up when performing the hamstring flexibility test), then perform Knee Extension (page 242) until you have full range of motion in the hamstring. At this time stop strengthening the quads and start strengthening the hamstrings using the Hamstring Curl.

Possibility 3: Strained Quad Causing Shortened Hamstring

Just as a strain of the hamstrings can have an effect on the position of the pelvis and the length of the lower back muscles, so can a strained quad. If the quad strains, this will decrease the force that helps oppose the force created by the hamstring. This causes the hamstring to shorten. Since the hamstring attaches to the back of the pelvis, if it shortens, it will pull the back of the pelvis down. This will cause an increased separation between the bottom of the back rib cage and the top of the pelvis. Since the lower back muscles (QLs) attach from the bottom of the rib cage to the top of the pelvis, the increased space between these landmarks will cause the lower back muscles to be overstretched. Once overstretched, they lose their ability to support the torso. Thus they strain and emit pain at the lower back.

To see if a strained quad is your problem, you will do a flexibility test, a muscle test, a posture analysis, and palpation.

Flexibility Test: First, you'll want to look at the flexibility of the quad and hamstring on the side where you are experiencing lower back pain.

To test the quad's flexibility, stand holding on to a sturdy object with one hand and then grab the ankle of the leg on the side you are experiencing pain. Try to pull your ankle to your buttocks. If you can, you have full range of motion, which indicates that the quads are at their proper length.

Now test your hamstring. Lie on your back, bending the knee on the side where you're not experiencing pain and keeping the foot of that leg on the floor. Have somebody try to raise your other leg—the leg on the side where you're experiencing pain—with the knee straight. You should be able to raise your leg so it is pointing straight up. This is considered normal range of motion of the hamstring. If you cannot do this, you have a tight, shortened hamstring. This indicates the quad is strained.

Muscle Testing: Next, we can look at muscle strength of the quad and hamstring on the side where you are experiencing pain.

To do this, sit on a sturdy chair. You will need somebody to help you test your strength. You will do the testing on the side experiencing the pain while keeping the other foot on the floor. While sitting, lift the foot on the painful side off the floor with the knee bent to about 70 degrees. Your helper will place one hand on the top of the thigh and one in front of the ankle. You will try to extend the knee while the person tries to stop you at the ankle. This is the test for quad strength. Now have the person take his or her hand and put it behind the ankle. From the same start position as before (the knee bent to 70 degrees), try to bend your knee more while the person tries to stop you. This is how you test the strength of the hamstrings. If the kicking forward is weaker than the pulling backward, this is another indication that the strained hamstring is causing the lower back pain. You may also find that pain is elicited either at the front of the thigh or at the knee because of the quad strain. This would only corroborate this diagnosis even more.

Posture Analysis: Next, we can look at posture. Looking at yourself from the side in a mirror, note the position of your pelvis. To do this, you will identify the ASIS and the PSIS (see page 126 if you need more information on this) and look to see if they are even. Do this on one side and then the other. If you find that the PSIS is lower than the ASIS on the side with lower back pain and this tilt is greater than on the unaffected side, this indicates a strained quad. You will also notice a more pronounced flattening of the lower back on the painful side.

Palpation: Finally, we can look to palpation. Feel along the quad muscles and the associated tendons that attach to the knee. See if you can find knots or locations of pain along the muscle and tendons. Compare how the quads feel on the side with lower back pain with how the quads feel on the unaffected side.

You'll also want to palpate your lower back; you'll need someone to help you with this. First, lie on your stomach and have your helper feel the lower back region on the side where you are having pain. Feel for the lower back muscles, the quadratus lumborum. Have your helper press down on this muscle along its whole length, from the point where it attaches to the rib cage to where it attaches to the pelvis.

Finding the knotting in the quads and the knotting and pain elicited in the lower back muscles reinforces the diagnosis that your one-sided lower back pain is due to a strained hamstring.

If the cause of your pain is a strained quad and a shortened hamstring, the key to resolving the pain is to stretch the hamstrings and strengthen the quads, glutes, and hip abductors on the side where you are experiencing pain. The exercises to be performed are:

1. Hamstring Stretch (page 248)
2. Calf Stretch (page 247)
3. Squats (page 245) or Lunges (page 243) or Leg Press (page 243)
4. Knee Extension (page 242)
5. Hip Extension (page 242)
6. Hip Abduction (page 241)

Possibility 4: Deficit of Single-Sided Hip, Knee, or Ankle Musculature

There is one other option of a cause for pain in one side of the back: an injury of the hip, knee, or ankle. If none of the scenarios I have identified above seem to fit your situation, I want you to think about whether you had an injury, be it a strain, a sprain, or even a prior surgery, to your hip, knee, or ankle. If the strength of the musculature at these locations did not return to full capacity, then a deficit of strength remains. Since your body weight is transmitted from your torso to the hip, the knee, the ankle, and the foot, any lost strength along the way could cause the lower back muscles to overwork and strain, emitting pain at the lower back.

I actually had a patient who had lower back pain on one side of his back. In evaluating him I found that he had a weak ankle on the side opposite his pain. When I asked him about this, he told me that he had broken his ankle a couple of years earlier. He had forgotten about the injury and never considered it a possible cause of his lower back pain. I ended up focusing most of my treatment on the injured ankle and lower extremity musculature. Within a couple of weeks, his lower back pain was resolved. The key in this case was to recognize that a previous injury altered his ability to bear weight, which caused his lower back muscles to overwork, strain, and emit pain at the lower back. If it appears that the cause of your lower back pain may be due to a prior injury somewhere else in the body, try to evaluate that area by performing the tests in the chapter that pertains to that region. Hopefully you can identify the cause of this prior injury and resolve it so the lower back can function normally.

CHAPTER 8

THE
GLUTEAL
REGION

MUSCULATURE OF THE GLUTEAL REGION

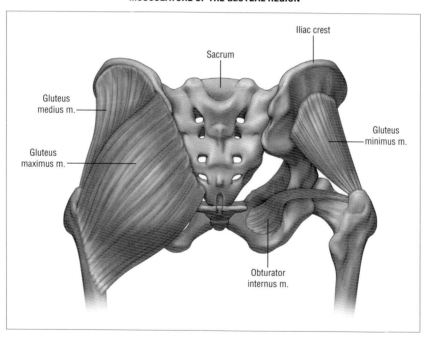

Sacrum

Iliac crest

Gluteus
medius m.

Gluteus
minimus m.

Gluteus
maximus m.

Obturator
internus m.

DEEP MUSCLES OF THE GLUTEAL REGION

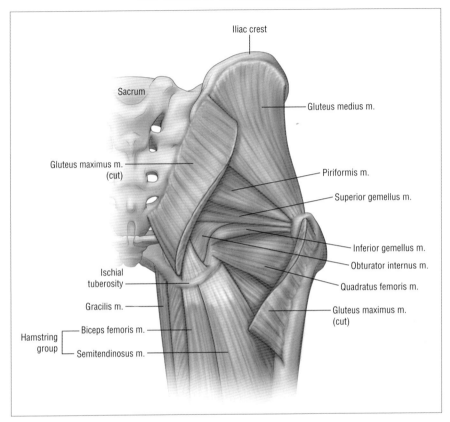

Pain at the gluteal region seems to be the most misunderstood of anywhere in the body simply because of its proximity to the lower back. Most medical practitioners simply group pain in this region with pain at the lumbar region. The patients themselves don't understand the distinction either. Over 20 years, whenever I ended up finding a problem with the gluteal region, the evaluations would typically start the same: I would ask where they were experiencing pain. They would tell me it was at their lower back. They would go on to say they'd had an MRI that showed a herniated disc, stenosis, or a nerve root impingement. Then I would ask them to point to where their pain was, and inevitably they would point to the gluteal region.

Because of this common misunderstanding, I would like to start this chapter by explaining the basic parameters of the region. The delineating line between the lower back and the gluteal region is the pelvic rim (iliac crest). Most people perceive this as their hips. Put your hands on your hips with your thumbs in the back. Now imagine a line running across the back of your body from thumb to thumb. This is the separating line between the lower back and the gluteal region. If your pain is below this line, your pain is in the gluteal region, so please work through the suggestions in this chapter. If your pain is above the line, it is in the lower back, so address your pain as noted in Chapter 7.

Let's be very clear: if your pain is found to be in the gluteal region and you are being told that this pain is coming from a structure in the lumbar region, such as a herniated disc, stenosis, or a pinched nerve, there is no way that this diagnosis can be correct. There is no nerve that connects between the lumbar spine and the gluteal region. Nerves that innervate the tissues of the gluteal region stem from the sacral spine.

PAIN IN THE GLUTEAL REGION (NO SCIATICA)

When looking at the gluteal region, what must first be understood is that all the muscles in the region attach from the hip joint to the pelvis or sacral spine. The most superficial muscle group that covers the region is the gluteus maximus muscle. This muscle helps you stand upright. To the side of the gluteal region just above the hip joint itself is the gluteus medius. This is the muscle most critical to supporting you and providing balance when you are standing on a single leg. Below and deeper than the gluteus maximus is a group of muscles responsible for rotating the hip joint, which basically means turning your foot in and out. One of these muscles is the piriformis, which attaches from the sacral spine bones, runs diagonally across the gluteal region, and attaches at the hip joint.

It's important to understand the relationship between the muscles of the gluteal region and the hip because many of the clinical indicators that point to a muscular cause for pain in the gluteal region are related to hip function. And for the most part, pain in the gluteal region develops because of a strained piriformis.

Generally a strain in the piriformis muscle comes because of a weakness in the glute med. Both muscles play a role in stabilizing the hip joint and pelvis during movement—at that point when you're standing on one leg when walking.

When you walk, you take one foot off the ground to place it in front of you to create forward motion. While you are standing on one leg, your pelvis must be level. If it does not stay level while your weight is on one leg, the hip on the opposite side can drop, which creates a decrease in the space between the hip and the ground. What this means is that there is less space for the leg that is in motion to pass through, and often the foot catches on its way to the front, making you susceptible to tripping. Your balance will also be thrown off because your center of mass will begin to shift toward the opposite side from which you are standing. This makes it more likely that you'll fall to the side. The glute med and the piriformis both work to make sure the pelvis stays level so neither of these things happens. The glute med is in the best position to achieve these goals. If the glute med strains because it does not have the strength to perform these tasks, the piriformis will try to compensate, which leads to it straining and emitting pain at the gluteal region on the same side as the glute med strain.

Before we jump into the tests, I'd like to explain why the glute med on one side can cause a strained piriformis on the other. If the glute med strains, the lower back muscles on the opposite side try to compensate. This will cause a strain in the lower back muscles, which leads to them shortening, causing the hip on the opposite side from the strained glute med to be elevated. With this shift, there is a leg length discrepancy. On the side with the higher hip, there is too much distance between the pelvis and the floor, and each step on this side requires you to step down farther every time you take a step. This means that an excessive force must be absorbed with each step. The piriformis tries to absorb this force but eventually strains and emits pain at the gluteal region on the opposite side of the glute med strain.

To find out if your gluteal pain is coming from a strained piriformis—along with which glute med led to the piriformis strain—you will do posture analysis, a single leg standing test, a muscle test, and some palpation.

Posture Analysis: The first test we can look at is hip height. Stand in front of a mirror that can provide a full view of you from the front. Place your hands on the rim of your pelvis (most people consider this their hips) and see if one hand is higher than the other. If the hip is higher on the same side as your pain, this indicates that the glute med on the opposite side of your body is strained. If the hip is higher on the opposite side of your body from the pain, this indicates that the glute med on the same side as the pain is strained.

Single Leg Standing Test: The next test to look at is the single leg standing test. Try to stand on one leg and then try to stand on the other. If one leg is more difficult to stand on, this indicates a strained glute med. Note if the strain is on the same side as your gluteal pain or on the opposite side.

Muscle Testing: Another way to confirm a diagnosis of a strained glute med is to test the strength of your glute meds. To perform this test, you'll need the help of someone else. First, lie down on a firm surface on your side. Raise your top leg a few inches, so it runs parallel to the ground. Make sure to keep it in line with your torso, not drifting forward or backward. Have your helper place one hand on your pelvis just above the hip joint and the other on your ankle. Try to push up at the ankle while the person tries to stop you. Then turn over and try the same test with the other leg. If the glute med is weaker on the same side where you are having the gluteal pain, this indicates that the strained glute med is on the same side as your pain. If the glute med on the opposite side of your body is weaker, this is an indication of strain on the opposite side.

Palpation: Finally, we can do some palpation. Feel for the piriformis muscle where the pain is being experienced. See if you can find knots in the muscle and if you increase the pain in the gluteal region by pressing on them. This will indicate if the piriformis is the cause of your gluteal pain. Now feel for the glute med on both sides. See if you can find knots in this muscle or if pressing on it causes pain. The side where there are knots and pain is the side with the strained glute med that led to the strained piriformis.

In the case of treating gluteal region pain, the key is to strengthen the glute meds, gluteus maximus, and hamstrings and to stretch the piriformis muscle. While it may be obvious why we need to strengthen the glute med, we should work on the gluteus maximus and hamstrings because they are also integrally involved in support when standing on a single leg. They are both hip extensors, which help you stand upright. When you are standing upright optimally, the skeletal structure supports most of the body. This means muscles have to work less. When they work less, more energy can go toward the glute meds to help create the force necessary to sustain balance when single-leg standing.

As a general rule, I have found that there is no such thing as too much strength when it comes to the glute meds. So even if the gluteal region pain is created by one or the other glute med straining, I would suggest strengthening both glute meds. Start by strengthening only the weakened glute med first with the Hip Abduction exercise. Once the pain is resolved, then begin to strengthen the glute med on the opposite side to achieve maximal strength of the glute meds. Other than the Hip Abduction exercise, you will perform all of the following exercises only on the affected side:

1. Hip Abduction (page 241)
2. Hamstring Curl (page 240)
3. Hip Extension (page 242)
4. Straight Leg Deadlifts (page 246)
5. Piriformis Stretch (page 249)

PAIN IN THE GLUTEAL REGION (WITH SCIATICA)

PIRIFORMIS MUSCLE AND SCIATIC NERVE

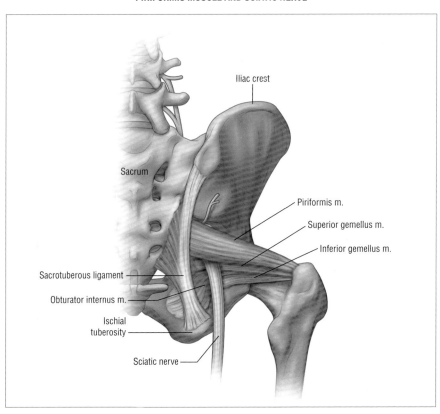

SCIATIC NERVE (NERVE ROOTS AND NERVE BEGINNING IN GLUTEAL REGION)

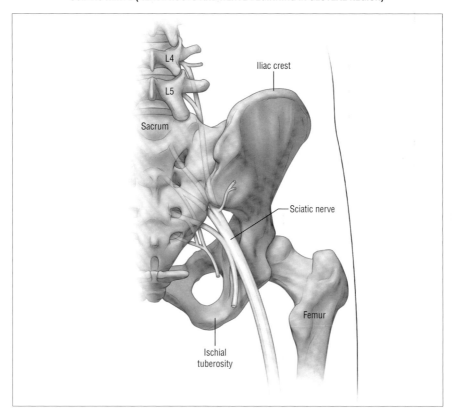

Before we get into the clinical indicators associated with sciatica, I want to discuss the existing viewpoint of the medical establishment regarding the cause of sciatica, which leads to way too many unnecessary back surgeries.

Sciatica creates pain spanning from the gluteal region down the back of the leg to the lower leg and, in most cases, to the foot. In medical school, I was taught that sciatica is associated with a herniated disc or stenosis in the lumbar spine that impinged on one of the seven nerve roots of the sciatic nerve. The claim is that the cause is not impingement of the nerve itself, just the nerve roots. The reason for this is that the roots are the only part of the nerve in contact with the lumbar spine.

However, the symptoms that would be associated with a nerve root impingement don't match the symptoms of sciatica. The nerve roots send signals to specific areas of the skin, known as dermatomes. If a nerve root were impinged, the pain would be felt in that area of the skin, not along the entire length of the sciatic nerve. For instance, if there was an impingement of the L4 (the fourth lumbar vertebrae) nerve root, symptoms should be experienced mostly at the inner shin. If there were impingement of the L5 nerve root, pain would occur at the outer shin. To cause the symptoms of sciatica, all the sciatic nerve roots would have to be impinged.

DERMATOMAL CHART OF LEGS AND GLUTEAL REGION

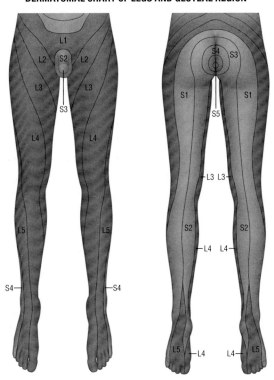

Impingement of the sciatic nerve itself makes sense with the symptoms of sciatica. The sciatic nerve runs from the gluteal region to the back of the knee, passing in extremely close proximity to the piriformis muscle. (In fact, in 30 percent of the population, the sciatic nerve actually passes through the piriformis muscle.) With this proximity, a strained piriformis muscle can impinge on the sciatic nerve. This is what I've found over 20 years of practice—that the strained piriformis is pinching the sciatic nerve. Remember the study we talked about in

Chapter 2 in which Dr. Aaron Filler confirmed that 93 percent of sciatica cases are the result of a strained piriformis muscle impinging on the sciatic nerve in the gluteal region?

The question is why would the piriformis strain in the first place? The answer is that the piriformis—along with the glute med—is a pelvic stabilizing muscle. This means that it helps support the pelvis while the muscles that create motion, such as the quads and hamstrings, pull from the pelvis to move the knee. If the glute med strains, the piriformis tries to compensate but eventually strains as well, creating the possibility of thickening and impinging on the sciatic nerve. At the gluteal region, there is a hierarchy of how the muscles strain from superficial to deep. Since the piriformis is the deepest muscle, it is the last muscle to attempt to perform its functional task before straining.

Gluteal pain on one side with sciatica can be caused by a strained glute med on either side of the body—just as with gluteal pain without sciatica.

If the glute med strains, the lower back muscles on the opposite side try to compensate. This will cause a strain in the lower back muscles, which leads them to shorten and pull up the hip on the opposite side from the strained glute med. With this shift, there is a leg length discrepancy. On the side with the higher hip, there is too much distance between the pelvis and the floor, and each step on this side requires you to step down farther every time you take a step. This means that an excessive force must be absorbed with each step. The piriformis tries to absorb this force but eventually strains and emits pain at the gluteal region on the opposite side of the glute med strain.

To see if your gluteal pain with sciatica is coming from a strained piriformis muscle—along with which glute med led to the piriformis strain—you will do posture analysis, a single leg standing test, a muscle test, and some palpation.

Posture Analysis: First, you'll look at hip height. Stand in front of a mirror that can provide a full view of you from the front. Place your hands on the rim of your pelvis (most people consider this their hips) and see if one hand is higher than the other. If the hip on the same side as your sciatic pain is higher, this indicates a strained glute med on the opposite side of your body. If the hip on the opposite side as your sciatic pain is higher, this indicates a strain of the glute med on the same side.

Single Leg Standing Test: The next test to look at is the single leg standing test. Try to stand on one leg and then try to stand on the other. If one leg is more difficult to stand on, this indicates a strained glute med. Note if the strain is on the same side as your sciatic pain or on the opposite side.

Muscle Testing: Next, you can test the strength of your glute meds. To perform this test, you'll need the help of someone else. First, lie down on a firm surface on your side. Raise your top leg a few inches, so it runs parallel to the ground. Make sure to keep it in line with your torso, not drifting forward or backward. Have your helper place one hand on your pelvis just above the hip joint and the other on your ankle. Try to push up at the ankle while the person tries to stop you. Then turn over and try the same test with the other leg. If the glute med is weaker on the same side where you are having the sciatic pain, this indicates that the strained glute med is on the same side as your pain. If the glute med on the opposite side of your body is weaker, this is an indication of strain on the opposite side.

Palpation: Finally, we can do some palpation. Feel for the piriformis muscle where the pain is being experienced. See if you can find knots in the muscle and if you increase the sciatic pain. This will indicate if the piriformis is strained and impinging on your sciatic nerve. Now feel for the glute med on both sides. See if you can find knots in this muscle or if pressing on it causes an increase in the sciatic pain. The side where there are knots and pain is the side with the strained glute med that led to the strained piriformis.

If you are suffering from sciatic symptoms, then there is a two-step process that must be performed to resolve the symptoms. The process is different if the symptoms are the result of a glute med strain on the same side or the opposite side from the symptoms.

If the sciatic symptoms are found to be caused by a strained glute med on the same side as the pain, the key to resolving the symptoms is to strengthen the glute med, the quads, the gluteus maximus, and the anterior tibialis muscle (front shin muscle). While it is likely clear why you need to strengthen the glute med, strengthening the quads and anterior tibialis is important because this causes deactivation of the nerves that send signals to the posterior leg and gluteal region muscles, causing a shutting down of the sciatic nerve.

By following this process, you should reach the point where you are no longer getting sciatic symptoms anymore, but you will most likely still be getting pain in the gluteal region. Once this has been achieved, switch the exercises from the quads and anterior tibialis to strengthen the hamstrings and calves. This switch is designed to strengthen the muscles that work in conjunction with the glute med in order to prevent further straining that might then strain the piriformis, causing it to impinge on the sciatic nerve. The exercises you'll do initially to follow this process are the following, which should be performed on the side of the body where you are experiencing pain:

1. Piriformis Stretch (page 249)

2. Hip Abduction (page 241)

3. Knee Extension (page 242)

4. Dorsiflexion (page 240)

5. Hip Extension (page 242)

Once the sciatic symptoms have resolved, switch to the following (done on the side where you are experiencing pain):

1. Hip Abduction (page 241)

2. Hamstring Curl (page 240)

3. Standing Calf Raises (page 246)

4. Hip Extension (page 242)

5. Straight Leg Deadlifts (page 246)

If the glute med is strained on the opposite side from the sciatic symptoms, then the sciatic symptoms must be seen as secondary to the strain of the glute med. The focus of the strengthening through Hip Abduction must be focused on the opposite glute med. You will also stretch the piriformis on the same side of the sciatic symptoms. By strengthening the glute med on the opposite side from the sciatic symptoms, the trauma of the excessive load caused by the strain is resolved. This prevents the piriformis from having to absorb the shock from the increased length of the step-down on the side of the symptoms. This stops the piriformis from straining, which means that it will not impinge on the sciatic nerve, thus resolving the sciatic symptoms. Once the sciatica resolves, you will be left with pain in the gluteal region only. Once you get to this point, you can strengthen the gluteus maximus, hamstrings, and calves on the side where the sciatic symptoms were occurring. This will help strengthen the muscles that work in conjunction with the glute med and the piriformis to help support you and prevent the piriformis from straining and impinging on the sciatic nerve.

In this case, the exercises to perform to resolve the symptoms initially are:

1. Hip Abduction on the side opposite the sciatic symptoms (page 241)
2. Piriformis Stretch on the same side (page 249)

Once the sciatic symptoms have resolved, then perform these exercises on the side where you are experiencing pain:

1. Hamstring Curl (page 240)
2. Standing Calf Raises (page 246)
3. Hip Extension (page 242)
4. Straight Leg Deadlifts (page 246)

CHAPTER 9

THE
KNEE

MUSCLES OF THE LATERAL KNEE

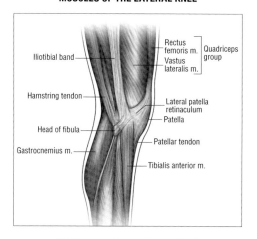

Iliotibial band

Rectus femoris m.
Vastus lateralis m.
} Quadriceps group

Hamstring tendon

Lateral patella retinaculum

Patella

Head of fibula

Patellar tendon

Gastrocnemius m.

Tibialis anterior m.

POSTERIOR MUSCLES OF THE KNEE

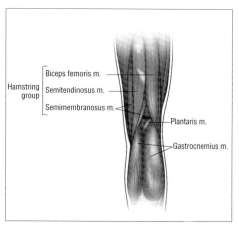

Hamstring group {
Biceps femoris m.
Semitendinosus m.
Semimembranosus m.

Plantaris m.

Gastrocnemius m.

ANTERIOR MUSCLES OF THE KNEE

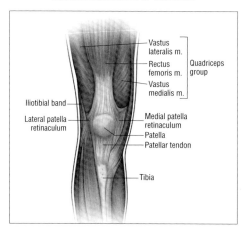

Vastus lateralis m.
Rectus femoris m.
Vastus medialis m.
} Quadriceps group

Iliotibial band

Lateral patella retinaculum

Medial patella retinaculum

Patella

Patellar tendon

Tibia

BONY ANATOMY OF THE KNEE

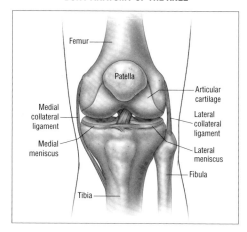

Femur

Patella

Articular cartilage

Medial collateral ligament

Lateral collateral ligament

Medial meniscus

Lateral meniscus

Fibula

Tibia

The knee is a unique joint because it is not only the joint where locomotion takes place but also the joint from which we get most of our ability to bend. Because we need both strength enough to move us forward and enough range of motion to allow us to bend, the joint of the knee needs both stability and mobility. This dual need brings with it some interesting structural intricacies. Basically the knee joint is not just one joint, it's two: the joint between the thigh bone (femur) and the lower leg bone (tibia) and the joint between the thigh bone (femur) and the kneecap (patella).

The joint between the thigh bone and the lower leg bone is where stability comes from. This joint allows you to transmit weight from the upper body and torso to the ground. The joint between the kneecap and the thigh bone is where power is created and movement is formed.

The quad (front thigh muscle) is connected to the kneecap via a tendon. The kneecap is then connected to the lower leg bone via another tendon. It is the quad that actually moves the lower leg to bend the knee or swings the lower leg forward, as with walking.

It is critical to understand that pain can occur at either of these two joints; thus it is essential to determine which is emitting the pain. A diagnosis can easily be disputed if the structure being diagnosed as the cause of pain is not located where the pain is being elicited. The best example of this is the diagnosis of a meniscus tear identified on an MRI. Many people with this diagnosis experience pain between the thigh bone and kneecap, which is not where it would be expected. Pain should be experienced at the joint line between the thigh bone and lower leg bone.

It is also possible to have pain from irritated fat pads that sit under the kneecap. If you have an occupation or hobby where you are on your knees a lot, it is possible to irritate the fat pads enough that they emit pain. Curing this irritation can only happen if the scar tissue at the fat pads is massaged out. Osgood–Schlatter disease is a condition that can also cause knee pain. This is associated with a growth spurt in adolescents, in which the bones grow quickly. Since muscles are attached to these bones, the muscles are lengthened quickly as well. This can cause the muscles to lose their ability to create force and thus cause pain at the knee. This pain can often be corrected by muscle-strengthening exercises; however, I will not be covering those in this book.

In this chapter you will find a description of the most common causes of knee pain, along with clinical tests to confirm which muscle is emitting the pain. Once you have determined where the pain is coming from, please go to the Appendix to learn the muscle-strengthening exercises that will help resolve your pain.

PAIN IN BOTH KNEES

While I am discussing pain in both knees in this section, please keep in mind that I am not talking about pain that began in one knee and then later came into the other knee. Here we are talking about pain in both knees that resulted from a singular cause.

If the pain started in both knees at the same time, the most likely cause of this is a posture called forward center of mass. Forward center of mass is when the bulk of your weight is aligned in front of your ankles, as if you're constantly leaning forward from the ankles. This occurs in most cases because there is a muscle imbalance between the hip flexors and quads (front-of-body muscles) versus the glutes and hamstrings (back-of-body muscles).

POSTURE ANALYSIS—NORMAL

POSTURE ANALYSIS—FORWARD CENTER OF MASS

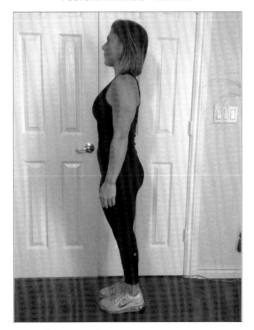
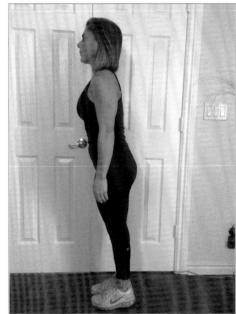

Because most of the work your muscles do happens in front of you (walking, climbing, and so on), the muscles in the front of your body get worked more and strengthen more. This makes them shorten, which pulls you forward at the hip joint. In turn, this shifts your weight in front of your ankles, creating an increased load on your knee joints when standing or walking. This increased load manifests in more extension, or straightening, through the knee when the leg is fully straightened. This causes compression of the kneecap, which creates irritation and pain.

To verify that your pain is coming from a forward center of mass posture, you will perform a number of clinical tests, including an analysis of posture, muscle testing, and flexibility testing.

Posture Analysis: The first test to confirm this diagnosis is a postural evaluation. Stand (as you would normally) with your side facing a mirror. Look at your ear in relationship to your ankle. If your ear aligns with the middle or front of your foot versus your ankle, this is the first indication that forward center of mass is the cause of your knee pain.

Try to feel where you support weight on your foot. Standing as you would normally stand, try to feel if you are weight bearing more on the balls of the feet, the heel, or evenly between the two. If the bulk of your weight is on the balls of your feet, this reinforces the idea that you have a forward center of mass.

Muscle Testing: To do this, sit on a sturdy chair. You will need somebody to help you test your strength. You will be sitting with one foot on the floor and one foot off the floor with the knee bent to about 70 degrees. The person will place one hand on the top of the thigh and one in front of the ankle. You will try to extend the knee while the person tries to stop you at the ankle. This is the test for quad strength. Now have the person take his or her hand and put it behind the ankle. From the same start position as before (the knee bent to 70 degrees), try to bend your knee more while the person tries to stop you. This is how you test the strength of the hamstrings. If the kicking out is stronger than the pulling backward, this is another confirming indicator that forward center of mass could be your problem. You will want to do this test on both sides of the body to confirm the muscle imbalance on both sides.

Flexibility Testing: Finally, you can look at flexibility of the quads and hamstrings. To test the quads' flexibility, stand holding on to a sturdy object with one hand and then grab the ankle of the leg on the other side. Try to pull your ankle to your buttocks. If you can't reach your heel to your buttocks while also keeping your knee slightly behind the hip, then your quads are tight.

Now test your hamstrings. Lie on your back with one knee bent and the foot of that leg on the floor. Have somebody try to raise your other leg with the knee straight. You should be able to raise your leg so it is pointing straight up. This is considered normal range of motion of the hamstrings. If you cannot do this, you have a tight hamstring.

If both the quads and hamstrings are tight, this is the final indication that your knee pain is being caused by a forward center of mass.

To resolve the muscle imbalances that account for forward center of mass, you'll want to do the following strengthening and stretching exercises on both sides of the body:

1. Quad Stretch (page 249)
2. Hip Flexor Stretch (page 248)
3. Hamstring Curl (page 240)
4. Straight Leg Deadlifts (page 246)
5. Hip Extension (page 242)
6. Hip Abduction (page 241)
7. Dorsiflexion (page 240)

PAIN IN A SINGLE KNEE

Possibility 1: Muscle Imbalance Between Quads and Hamstrings

This is by far the most common cause of pain in a single knee. Because most of our action takes place in front of our bodies (walking, climbing stairs, and so on), the quads are used more than the hamstrings, and as a result, they become stronger than the hamstrings. If this muscle imbalance increases enough, the quads shorten because of the lack of equally opposing force from the hamstrings. Since the quads are attached to the kneecap, the shortened quads will pull the kneecap up and cause it to be compressed in the knee joint. This causes irritation and pain around the kneecap.

To verify that your pain is coming from a muscle imbalance between the quads and hamstrings, you will do flexibility testing, muscle testing, palpation, and a movement called the patella glide.

Flexibility Testing: First, you will test the flexibility of the quads in both legs in order to do a comparison.

To test the quads' flexibility, stand holding on to a sturdy object or wall with one hand and then grab the ankle of the leg on the other side. Try to pull your ankle to your buttocks. If you can't reach your heel to your buttocks while also keeping your knee slightly behind your hip, then your quads are tight. Now test the other side.

If the quad on the side where you are experiencing knee pain is shorter than the unaffected side, this is the first positive sign that the cause of the knee pain is a muscle imbalance between the quads and hamstrings.

Muscle Testing: The next test is muscle testing the quads and hamstrings of both legs. Again, we're trying to create a comparison between the strength of the muscles in the painful knee versus the not-painful knee.

To do this, sit on a sturdy chair. You will need somebody to help you test your strength. You will be sitting with the foot on the same side as the painful knee on the floor and the other foot off the floor with the knee bent to about 70 degrees. Your helper will place one hand on the top of the thigh and one in front of the ankle. You will try to extend the knee while the person tries to stop you at the ankle. Once you have tested this quad, alternate the position to test the other leg. Notice if the quad associated with your painful knee is weaker or about the same as the unaffected knee.

Next, you will compare the strength of the hamstrings. Again switch legs, placing the foot on the same side as your pain on the floor. Lift the other foot off the floor with the knee bent to about 70 degrees. This time, have your helper place one hand on the top of the thigh and one behind the ankle. Now try to bend your knee more while the person tries to stop you. Do this again with the other leg and notice if one leg is stronger than the other.

If you find that the quad strength is about the same or just slightly weaker on the side with the knee pain, but the hamstring of that leg is noticeably weaker, this is another indication that an imbalance between the quads and the hamstrings could be causing your knee pain.

Palpation: The next test to be performed is palpation. Remember, the goal of palpation is to incite pain in order to identify which tissue is emitting pain. The bottom end of the femur is composed of two projections called femoral condyles—one on each side of the kneecap (see the illustration at the start of the chapter). To determine if the cause of the pain is a muscle imbalance between the quads and hamstrings, try to press on the space between the side of the kneecap and the femoral condyles. You want to try to press just to the sides of the kneecap—between the kneecap and the condyles on either side of the kneecap. Your leg should be in a relaxed position so the muscles are loose and the kneecap has no muscle tone against it. If pain is elicited when you press here, this is another confirming finding of this diagnosis.

Patella Glide: The final test to be performed to determine if a muscle imbalance is the cause of the knee region pain is what is known as a patella glide. This is where you try to move the kneecap side to side while sitting with your knee straight and your whole leg supported. This position will allow you to relax your quad, which is key when the patella is being tested. What you are looking for is to see how easy it is to move the kneecap. You will be checking both how easily and how far you can move the kneecap at the affected knee versus the unaffected knee. If a muscle imbalance exists between the quads and hamstrings, the quad will create severe upward force on the kneecap. This will make it much harder for the kneecap to be moved side to side, and the kneecap will also not move as far on the affected leg. This would be another indicator that a muscle imbalance is the cause of the knee region pain.

To resolve a muscle imbalance between the quads and the hamstrings, the key is to stretch the quads and strengthen the hamstrings and gastrocnemius portion of the calf. (The calf is composed of two muscles, the soleus and the gastrocnemius; the gastrocnemius passes over the knee joint while the soleus does not.) The exercises to be performed, only on the side where you are experiencing pain, are:

1. Quad Stretch (page 249)
2. Hamstring Curl (page 240)
3. Straight Leg Deadlifts (page 246)
4. Standing Calf Raises (page 246)
5. Hip Abduction (page 241)

Possibility 2: Quad Strain

A quad strain can alter the pull on the kneecap, just as happens with the muscle imbalance between the quad and the hamstring. With a strained quad there is a decrease in the upward force created on the kneecap. This will cause the kneecap to slightly rise or float in the knee joint. As the kneecap floats in the joint, it will be pulled toward the outside of the leg since most of the quad that creates the pull on the kneecap sits more to the outside of (lateral to) the knee joint. This movement of the kneecap will create a situation where the kneecap can now impact the lateral border of the knee joint. This increased force between the kneecap and the lateral border of the knee joint will cause irritation and pain at the kneecap region.

To verify that your pain is coming from a quad strain, you will do flexibility testing, muscle testing, palpation, and a movement called the patella glide.

Flexibility Testing: The first test to confirm this as the cause of knee region pain is testing the flexibility of your hamstrings. We will do this on both the side with pain and the one without in order to create a comparison.

Lie on your back with one knee bent and the foot of that leg on the floor. Have somebody try to raise your other leg with the knee straight. Then switch sides, trying to raise the other leg.

If the hamstrings on the side where you are experiencing knee pain are shorter, this is the first positive sign that the cause of the knee pain is a quad strain.

Muscle Testing: Next, muscle test the quads and hamstrings of both legs. Again, we're trying to create a comparison between the strength of the muscles associated with the painful knee versus the not-painful knee.

To do this, sit on a sturdy chair. You will need somebody to help you test your strength. You will be sitting with the foot on the same side as the painful knee on the floor and the other foot off the floor with the knee bent to about 70 degrees. Your helper will place one hand on the top of the thigh and one in front of the ankle. You will try to extend the knee while the person tries to stop you at the ankle. Once you have tested this quad, alternate the position to test the other leg. Notice if the quad associated with your painful knee is weaker or about the same as the unaffected knee.

Next, you will compare the strength of the hamstrings. Again switch legs, placing the foot on the same side as your pain on the floor. Lift the other foot off the floor with the knee bent to about 70 degrees. This time, have your helper place one hand on the top of the thigh and one behind the ankle. Now try to bend your knee more while the person tries to stop you. Do this again with the other leg and notice if one leg is stronger than the other.

If you find that the quad strength is decreased in the leg with the knee pain and the strength of the hamstrings is about the same on both sides, this is the next indication that a quad strain is causing your pain.

Palpation: The next test to be performed is palpation. Remember, the goal of palpation is to incite pain in order to identify which tissue is emitting pain. The bottom end of the femur is composed of two projections called femoral condyles—one on each side of the kneecap (see the illustration at the start of the chapter). To determine if the cause of the pain is a quad strain, try to press just the sides of the kneecap in the space between the side of the kneecap and the femoral condyles. Your leg should be in a relaxed position so the muscles are loose and the kneecap has no muscle tone against it. If pain is elicited when you press here, this is another confirmation of this diagnosis.

Patella Glide: The final test to be performed is the patella glide. This is where you try to move the kneecap side to side with your knee straight and your whole leg supported. This position will allow you to relax your quad, which is key when the patella is being tested. What you are looking for is to see how easy it is to move the kneecap. You will be checking both how easily and how far you can move the kneecap at the affected knee versus the unaffected knee. An increased ease in moving the kneecap side to side at the affected knee is another indicator that a quad strain is the cause of your knee pain.

To resolve the symptoms of a quad strain, the key is to stretch the hamstrings and calf and strengthen the quads and anterior tibialis (front shin muscle). The exercises to be performed, only on the side of the affected knee, are:

1. Hamstring Stretch (page 248)
2. Calf Stretch (page 247)
3. Squats (page 245) or Lunges (page 243) or Leg Press (page 243)
4. Dorsiflexion (page 240)
5. Hip Abduction (page 241)

Possibility 3: Strained Glute Med Causing Iliotibial Band (ITB) Strain

A strained gluteus medius (glute med) causing the iliotibial band (ITB) to strain is a somewhat less frequent cause of pain at the knee, oftentimes seen with runners.

The glute med plays a pivotal role in supporting you, especially when you stand on one leg, as in the case of walking or running. The glute med keeps the pelvis level when you are standing on one leg so balance is maintained. And with a strong glute med, the weight of the body is positioned above the leg you are standing on. With running or jogging, the pressure on the glute med is increased substantially, and if the muscle is not strong enough to accept this increased load, other muscles try to compensate. However, if you have a weakened glute med, the weight will shift more toward the middle of your body, making balance more difficult.

The ITB is a long thick band of connective tissue that attaches to the knee joint/cap. At the top of the band is a muscle called the tensor fasciae latae. If this muscle strains because of the extra work it is doing to compensate for the glute med, it creates more of a load on the band, which then thickens and shortens. The shortened band then pulls the kneecap laterally, causing it to impact the lateral border of the knee joint excessively, bringing with it irritation and pain. With this deviation, you can experience pain either just at the joint around the kneecap or both around the kneecap and at the lateral aspect of the thigh where the ITB extends.

To verify that your pain is coming from a strained glute med, you will do posture analysis, muscle testing, palpation, and a single leg stand test.

Posture Analysis: The first test is to look at your hip height. Stand in front of a mirror that can provide a full view of you from the front. Place your hands on the rim of your pelvis (most people consider this their hips) and see if one hand is higher than the other. If the glute med is strained on the side of the knee with pain, you will see that the opposite hip is elevated. This is because the lower back muscles on the opposite side have tried to compensate for the weakened glute med. As a result, the lower back muscle shortens, pulling up your hip on the side opposite your knee with pain.

Muscle Testing: The next step is to test the strength of your glute meds. You will want to do this test on both sides of your body in order to compare the strength of the painful side with the unaffected side.

To perform this test, you'll need the help of someone else. First, lie down on a firm surface on the side that has the knee pain. Raise your top leg a few inches, so it runs parallel to the ground. Make sure to keep it in line with your torso, not drifting forward or backward. Have your helper place one hand on your pelvis, just above the hip joint, and the other on your ankle. Try to push up at the ankle while the person tries to stop you. Then turn over and try the same test with the other leg.

If the glute med of the leg with knee pain is weaker than the opposite leg, this is another indicator that this is the correct diagnosis.

Palpation: The next test is palpation. Remember, with this test we are trying to elicit pain by applying pressure.

Lie on your side opposite the knee with pain. Try to feel the glute med and see if you can find knots in it. Also see if you can create pain in the knotty locations you find. Now feel along the ITB. If the ITB has strained, it will not be hard to find places along its length that are thickened and painful to touch. If you can find knots and pain at the glute med and the ITB of the leg with the knee pain, these are indicators that this is the right diagnosis.

Single Leg Standing Test: The final test for confirming this diagnosis is the single leg standing test. Try to stand on one leg and then try to stand on the other leg. If it is more difficult to stand on the leg with the knee pain, this is another confirming test that the cause of the knee pain is a strained glute med causing the ITB to strain.

To resolve a strained glute med causing an ITB strain, the key is to stretch the ITB and strengthen the glute med, quad, and anterior tibialis. The exercises to be performed are:

1. ITB Stretch (page 248)
2. Hip Abduction in sidelying or with a cable machine (page 241)
3. Knee Extension (page 242)
4. Dorsiflexion (page 240)

Possibility 4: Strained Medial Hamstring

In some cases, pain in one knee could be caused by strained hamstring muscles. This is different from simply having a muscle imbalance where the quads are stronger than the hamstrings. In the case of the muscle imbalance, the pain would be felt around the kneecap. But in the case of a strained hamstring muscle, the pain would be found at the attachment of the hamstrings near the knee joint and/or at the hamstring muscle itself. The pain associated with a medial hamstring strain would be experienced close to where pain associated with a meniscal tear would occur. So it is critical to be able to identify the attachment point of the hamstring tendons (where the hamstring tendons attach to the bones of the knee) to differentiate a meniscal tear from a hamstring strain.

To verify that your pain is coming from a strained medial hamstring, you will do palpation, muscle testing, and flexibility testing.

Palpation: The first test to be utilized to confirm this diagnosis is palpation. Remember, with this test we are trying to create pain in order to identify which tissue is causing your knee pain. In this instance, locate the point where the medial hamstring tendon attaches to the knee. Having your knee slightly bent should help to separate the joint line of the knee from the attachment point of the medial hamstring tendon. This is called the pes anserinus. It is a little bump just below and toward the inside of the knee joint. Press on this spot. If you have pain there, this is a confirming sign.

Next, press along the hamstring tendon, moving back toward the hamstring itself, and note if there is pain on the tendon. Finally, press on the medial hamstring muscle itself. If the hamstring tendon strained and is emitting pain, it is only because the muscle strained as well. You should be able to find some knots and tender points in the medial hamstring muscle.

Muscle Testing: Next, muscle test the hamstrings. In this test, we're trying to create a comparison between the strength of the muscles associated with the painful knee versus the not-painful knee.

To do this, sit on a sturdy chair. You will need somebody to help you test your strength. You will be sitting with the foot on the same side as the painful knee on the floor and the other foot off the floor with the knee bent to about 70 degrees. To isolate the medial hamstrings from the whole hamstring muscle, turn your foot in when performing the test. Your helper will place one hand on the top of the thigh and one behind the ankle. Now try to bend your knee more while the person tries to stop you. Do this again with the other leg and notice if one leg is stronger than the other.

If the medial hamstrings are weaker on the side with knee pain, this is a sign that a strained medial hamstring may be the cause of your pain.

Along with weakness, pain may be experienced at the medial hamstring tendon and/or muscle. This will reinforce the diagnosis even more.

Flexibility Testing: The final test for this diagnosis is a flexibility test for the hamstrings. We will do this on both the side with pain and the one without in order to create a comparison.

Lie on your back with one knee bent and the foot of that leg on the floor. Have somebody try to raise your other leg with the knee straight while your foot is rotated outward. Then switch sides, trying to raise the other leg.

If the medial hamstrings on the side where you are experiencing knee pain are shorter, meaning that this leg cannot be raised as high, this reinforces that the medial hamstrings have strained and are creating the pain at the medial aspect of the knee joint.

To resolve a strained medial hamstring, the first thing to determine is if the strain is mild or severe. If the hamstring cannot be stretched to 90 degrees (the angle between the torso and the leg), then it is severe. If the hamstring can be stretched to 90 degrees, then it is a mild strain. If it is severe, first you need to lengthen the hamstrings by doing the following exercises:

FLEXIBILITY TEST—HAMSTRING

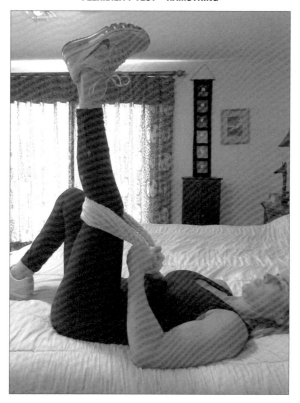

1. Knee Extension (page 242)

2. Dorsiflexion (page 240)

Once the hamstring can be stretched to 90 degrees, switch to:

1. Hamstring Curl (page 240)

2. Straight Leg Deadlifts (page 246)

3. Standing Calf Raises (page 246)

4. Hip Abduction (page 241)

If it is a mild strain, go directly to performing the Hamstring Curl, Straight Leg Deadlifts, Standing Calf Raises, and Hip Abduction on the side of the body where you are experiencing pain.

Possibility 5: Strained Gastrocnemius

As we start getting into these last few potential causes of knee pain, the pain that might be experienced is more likely at the muscle itself. There is, however, a chance that you'll experience pain at or near the attachment of these muscles to the knee joint.

The gastrocnemius is the part of the calf muscle that passes the back of the knee joint and attaches to the femur (thigh bone). In this particular case, you might feel pain at the back of the knee joint or from some portion of this muscle at the back of the lower leg up to and including the back of the knee joint.

The gastrocnemius will typically only strain if another muscle has strained first, causing it to take an additional load leading to a strain and emitting pain. The most likely muscle to strain and cause the gastrocnemius to overwork and strain is the gluteus medius muscle.

To verify that your pain is coming from a strained gastrocnemius muscle, you will do palpation and a single leg standing heel raise test.

Palpation: The first test to confirm that the cause of pain at the back of the knee is a strained gastrocnemius is palpation. To cause the gastrocnemius to be more prominent and easier to feel for, do this test with the knee extended, or straightened. Now feel behind the knee toward the sides of the joint. If the gastrocnemius is strained, you should be able to feel knotting and pain elicited on either side or both sides of the back of the knee. It is sometimes hard to differentiate between where the hamstring and the gastrocnemius muscles attach to the knee because they are very close together. To confirm that the gastrocnemius is the strained muscle and not the hamstrings, try to feel lower down on the muscle itself, from the attachment. You should be able to find more knotting in the main portion of the muscle.

Single Leg Standing Heel Raise Test: The other test is a single leg standing heel raise. If the gastrocnemius has strained, it will be more difficult to create a single leg heel raise because the calf muscle is responsible for creating this motion. First, stand on the leg without knee pain. Try to perform ten heel raises (moving from flat on your foot onto the balls of your foot) without touching the floor with the other foot. See how many you can do. Now try to perform a single leg heel raise with the leg with knee pain. See how many you can do. If you cannot do as many or you experience pain at the back of the knee or lower leg while performing this test, this is a positive indicator that a strained gastrocnemius is the cause of your knee pain.

FLEXIBILITY TEST—GASTROCNEMIUS

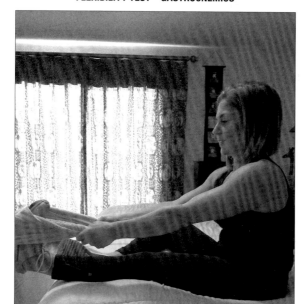

To resolve a gastrocnemius strain, first determine if the strain is mild or severe. To test this, sit down on the floor or another flat surface and extend one leg in front of you, keeping the other bent. (If this is uncomfortable or not possible, place a small pillow under the knee to keep the knee unlocked.) Place a towel around the balls of your foot (metatarsal heads) and pull the foot back toward you, stretching your calf muscle. Then switch legs and do the test again. If the affected leg is just as flexible as the unaffected leg, the strain is mild. If the affected leg is not as flexible, the strain is severe. If the strain is severe, start by performing the following exercises on the strained side:

1. Knee Extension (page 242)
2. Dorsiflexion (page 240)

Once the toes can be pulled back as far as the unaffected side, then switch to the following exercises:

1. Hamstring Curl only on the affected side (page 240)

2. Straight Leg Deadlifts only on the affected side (page 246)

3. Standing Calf Raises only on the affected side (page 246)

4. Hip Abduction on both sides (page 241)

If it is a mild strain, go directly to performing the Hamstring Curl, Straight Leg Deadlifts, Standing Calf Raises, and Hip Abduction.

Possibility 6: Strained Sartorius

MUSCLES OF THE THIGH—ANTERIOR VIEW

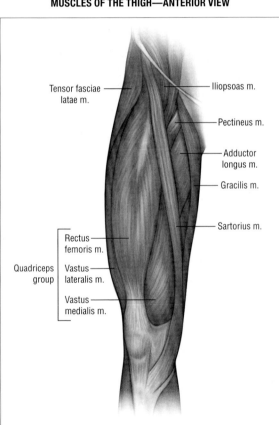

The sartorius is a muscle that attaches near the hip joint and follows along the inside of the front of the thigh and connects to the knee region at the same location as the inner hamstring tendon. If pain is felt at this location near the inside lower portion of the knee joint, called the pes anserinus, it is important to determine which muscle has strained so the right muscles can be treated. The sartorius is an important muscle to keep in mind because it has the ability to create pain at the groin region, the inner front thigh, or the inner knee. Remember, muscles that strain can create pain at their attachment points to bones or within the muscle itself.

The sartorius muscle tends to strain if the glute med has strained first. Because the sartorius runs on the inner side of the thigh, a strained glute med can cause it to shorten excessively, thus making it susceptible to straining. Most people who strain the sartorius muscle experience pain at its attachment point at the inside of the knee. There are three muscles that attach at this point, so it is important to determine which muscle has strained if pain is experienced at this location. In addition to having knee pain, people who have a strained sartorius also feel pain at the inner thigh.

To verify that your pain is coming from a strained sartorius muscle, you will do palpation and muscle testing.

Palpation: The first test to identify a strained sartorius as the cause of medial knee pain is palpation. Press along the muscle from one end to the other, making sure to press on its attachment at the inner lower knee region. If the sartorius has strained, you will typically have intense pain at this attachment point along with painful spots along the path of the muscle itself.

Muscle Testing: The next test is a muscle test, which will require someone to help you. To do this test, sit at the end of a surface with your lower legs hanging off from the knees. Your helper will place one hand on the top of the knee and one on the inner ankle. Then you will try to raise your knee up and out while simultaneously moving your ankle in toward the midline of the body. You will do this as your helper tries to resist your movement.

MUSCLE TESTING—SARTORIUS MUSCLE

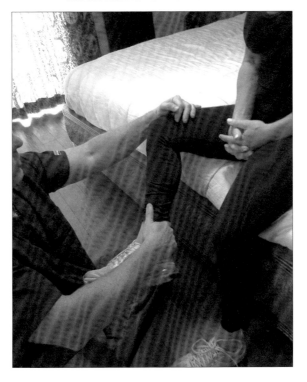

You will do this test first on the unaffected leg, then on the affected leg. Be sure that the resistance to moving the leg is performed correctly. While the hip flexor moves the knee up, the sartorius actually works when the knee is moving both up and out. If the leg with knee pain is weaker than the one without, or pain is elicited along the muscle or at its attachment at the knee during the test, this is an indication that you have a strained sartorius.

The final test to confirm this diagnosis is a strength test of the glute med. You will do this test on both sides of your body in order to compare the strength of the painful side with the unaffected side.

To perform this test, you'll need the help of someone else. First, lie down on a firm surface on the side that has the knee pain. Raise your top leg a few inches, so it runs parallel to the floor. Make sure to keep it in line with your torso, not drifting forward or backward. Have your helper place one hand on your pelvis, just above the hip joint, and the other on your ankle. Try to push up at the ankle while the person tries to stop you. Then turn over and try the same test with the other leg.

If the glute med of the leg with knee pain is weaker than the opposite leg, this reinforces the diagnosis of a strained sartorius as the cause of your knee pain.

To resolve a strained sartorius muscle, perform the following exercises on the side of your body with pain:

1. Sartorius Exercise (page 244)

2. Knee Extension (page 242)

3. Dorsiflexion (page 240)

4. Hip Abduction in sidelying or with a cable machine (page 241)

Possibility 7: Strained Gracilis

MUSCLES OF THE THIGH—ANTERIOR VIEW

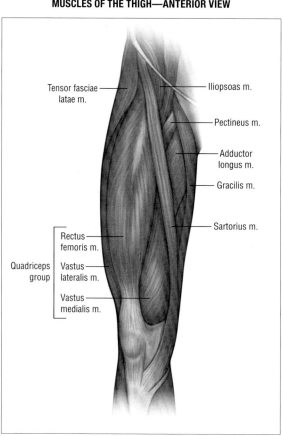

Tensor fasciae latae m.

Iliopsoas m.

Pectineus m.

Adductor longus m.

Gracilis m.

Sartorius m.

Rectus femoris m.

Quadriceps group

Vastus lateralis m.

Vastus medialis m.

The gracilis is the final muscle that attaches at the lower inner portion of the knee joint, known as the pes anserinus. This is a groin muscle that performs adduction, or pulling the legs together. It starts at the pubic bone near the groin and attaches at the knee.

A properly functioning glute med, which is an abductor muscle, is necessary to maintain proper posture and function. If it strains, the muscle that opposes it or performs the opposite action has a tendency to shorten—and one of those muscles is the gracilis, which is a strong adductor muscle. If an activity requires the legs to be spread apart for any distance, the gracilis has a strong chance of being overstretched and thus straining when it performs its function of pulling the legs back to center. When you see athletes straining their "groin" muscles, it is rarely because they are too weak. It is usually just the opposite: they are too strong in comparison to the hip abductors.

As a general rule, the adductor muscles are much stronger than the abductor muscles. This is why, as a general rule, I do not strengthen my patient's adductors without confirming that they are similar in strength to the abductor muscles.

To verify that your pain is coming from a strained gracilis muscle, you will do palpation and muscle testing.

Palpation: The first test to identify a strained gracilis as the cause of medial knee pain is palpation. Try to feel the muscle along its path all the way to its attachment at the inner lower knee region. If the gracilis has strained, you will typically have intense pain at its attachment near the knee joint along with painful spots along the path of the muscle.

Muscle Testing: Next, muscle test the gracilis muscle. You will need someone to help you perform this test. Lie down on a flat surface. Have your helper place one hand on the inside of your thigh just above the knee and one hand on the inside of the other ankle. He or she will try to stabilize the leg with the hand on the thigh while trying to pull the ankle away from the midline. You will try to resist the pressure being applied at your ankle.

MUSCLE TESTING—GRACILIS MUSCLE

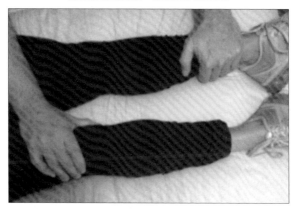

First, test the unaffected leg, pulling this ankle. Then test the affected leg. Make sure that when you are performing this test, the knee of the leg being tested is straight. If you are better able to resist the force of the ankle being pulled on the unaffected leg—and less able to resist on the affected leg—or if pain is elicited along the muscle or at its attachment at the knee on the affected leg, this is a sign that you might have a strained gracilis.

The final test to confirm this diagnosis is a strength test of the glute med. You will do this test on both sides of your body in order to compare the strength of the painful side with the unaffected side.

To perform this test, you'll need the help of someone else. First, lie down on a firm surface on the side that has the knee pain. Raise your top leg a few inches, so it runs parallel to the floor. Make sure to keep it in line with your torso, not drifting forward or backward. Have your helper place one hand on your pelvis, just above the hip joint, and the other on your ankle. Try to push up at the ankle while the person tries to stop you. Then turn over and try the same test with the other leg.

If the glute med of the leg with knee pain is weaker than the opposite leg, this reinforces the diagnosis of a strained gracilis muscle as the cause of your knee pain.

To resolve a strained gracilis muscle, perform the following exercises on the side where you are experiencing pain:

1. Gracilis Stretch (page 247)

2. Hip Abduction in sidelying or on a cable machine (page 241)

3. Knee Extension (page 242)

4. Dorsiflexion (page 240)

CHAPTER 10

THE
SHOULDER

BONY ANATOMY OF THE SHOULDER

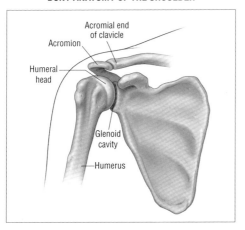

Acromial end
of clavicle

Acromion

Humeral
head

Glenoid
cavity

Humerus

BICEPS ATTACHMENT TO SHOULDER

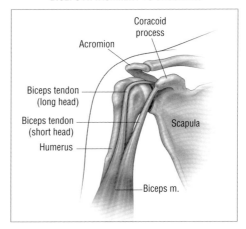

Coracoid
process

Acromion

Biceps tendon
(long head)

Biceps tendon
(short head)

Humerus

Scapula

Biceps m.

MUSCULATURE OF THE NECK AND UPPER BACK

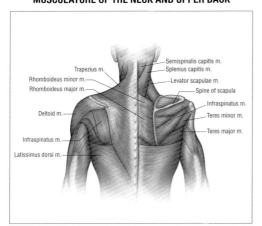

Trapezius m.

Rhomboideus minor m.
Rhomboideus major m.

Deltoid m.

Infraspinatus m.

Latissimus dorsi m.

Semispinalis capitis m.
Splenius capitis m.

Levator scapulae m.

Spine of scapula

Infraspinatus m.

Teres minor m.

Teres major m.

SERRATUS ANTERIOR MUSCLE

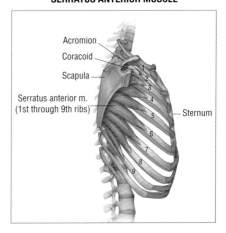

Acromion

Coracoid

Scapula

Serratus anterior m.
(1st through 9th ribs)

Sternum

1
2
3
4
5
6
7
8
9

The shoulder joint is composed of the upper arm bone joining with the end of the shoulder blade. In most joints, the motion happens because one bone of the joint moves around the other stable bone. For example, when bending the knee, the thigh bone is stable while the lower leg bone moves around it. In the shoulder, however, both bones move—the arm bone moves within the joint and at the same time the shoulder blade moves on the rib cage.

For this joint to work correctly—and to not hurt—the arm bone must move in a specific relationship to the shoulder blade. This relationship is referred to by a principle called the scapulohumeral rhythm, which states that for every two degrees of motion of the shoulder joint, the shoulder blade must move one degree. While the exact relationship is not important for you to understand, it does matter that you recognize that there is a relationship between the shoulder blade motion and shoulder motion. Associated with this is a relationship between the muscles that stabilize and move the shoulder blade and the muscles that stabilize and move the shoulder joint. As we discuss the muscular causes of shoulder joint pain, you will notice that in most cases the cause of the pain at the shoulder joint was created by a loss of the proper relationship between the muscles of the shoulder blade and the muscles of the shoulder joint.

In this chapter you will find a description of the muscle groups possibly involved in creating pain in your shoulder, along with clinical tests to confirm which muscle is emitting the pain. Once you have determined where the pain is coming from, please go to the Appendix to learn the muscle-strengthening exercises that will help resolve your pain.

PAIN IN THE FRONT OF THE SHOULDER

A rotator cuff strain causing shoulder impingement is by far the most common cause of shoulder region pain, and this pain is most often found in the front of the shoulder. The difference between the muscular cause of impingement syndrome and the structural cause promoted by physicians is that the muscular cause can be easily resolved and prevented from recurring by understanding the mechanism. The key to understanding what causes shoulder impingement syndrome is understanding the relationship between four muscles: (1) the muscles that move the shoulder joint, (2) the muscles that keep the upper arm bone in the shoulder joint when the shoulder moves, (3) the muscles that move the shoulder blade in synchrony with the shoulder joint, and (4) the muscles that keep the shoulder blade against the rib cage while it is moving.

Let's start by exploring the mechanics of the shoulder joint. As I mentioned, the shoulder joint is composed of the upper arm bone attaching at the end of the shoulder blade. As the arm is raised, the arm bone is stabilized in the joint at the end of the shoulder blade to create shoulder motion. At the same time the shoulder blade moves on the rib cage. For proper shoulder function to occur, you must have proper motion at the shoulder joint and proper motion of the shoulder blade moving on the rib cage.

Looking at the shoulder joint first, muscles like the deltoid have the ability to move the shoulder joint. The rotator cuff is a set of muscles associated with the shoulder that creates stability while allowing for range of motion. Because of the extreme range of motion required for normal function of the shoulder joint, little stability can be achieved through the use of ligaments and joint capsules. A unique method of providing stability was necessary for this joint. A dynamic stabilizer was needed to keep the arm bone in the shoulder joint while going through such a vast range of motion. The rotator cuff performs this function, and it is unique because the stability it provides is created by muscles, not ligaments. The rotator cuff muscles can constantly contract to achieve proper congruency between the arm bone and the shoulder joint during shoulder motion.

Another thing to note about the shoulder is that it is a distractive joint instead of a compressive joint, like the joints of the legs. What this means is that gravity is not forcing the joint surfaces together to provide stability. If you think about the knee, the weight of your body compresses the joint. This limits the extent that stability needs to be achieved through muscle or ligament. In the shoulder, however, the weight of the arm is pulling the two joint surfaces away from each other. This creates increased instability. This makes the job of the rotator cuff different from most muscles.

The next thing to understand is the acromion process, a small protrusion coming off the top of the end of the shoulder blade that makes up the superior border of the joint. As the arm is raised in the shoulder joint, the mechanics of the joint will cause the head of the upper arm bone to rise. If it rises enough, it can impact the acromion process; however, this should not happen if the muscles responsible for normal function are working properly. Between the acromion process and the head of the upper arm bone is a space known as the subacromial space. Running through this space are tendons. These include the biceps tendon and a couple of the rotator cuff tendons. If the shoulder isn't functioning correctly, the head of the upper arm bone can rise into the subacromial space and impinge on these tendons. The tendons then become irritated and emit pain, signaling that impingement has occurred. The tendon most associated with impingement syndrome due to a strained rotator cuff is the tendon of the long head of the biceps. This typically creates pain at the front of the shoulder.

Not only is the rotator cuff responsible for maintaining optimal congruency between the head of the upper arm bone and the shoulder joint, it must also pull down on the head of the upper arm bone as the arm is raised in the shoulder joint. By pulling down and keeping the head of the upper arm bone from rising, it prevents impingement of the space between the acromion process and the head of the upper arm bone.

Now that you understand how the rotator cuff affects the function of the shoulder joint, let's look at how other muscles can affect the health and well-being of the rotator cuff. For the rotator cuff to work correctly and create force from the shoulder blade on the head of the upper arm, the shoulder blade must be anchored to the rib cage. If the muscles responsible for anchoring the shoulder blade to the rib cage are not strong, the rotator cuff loses its ability to keep the arm bone in the shoulder joint. There are two main muscle groups responsible for stabilizing the shoulder blade against the rib cage. These are the serratus anterior and the muscles of the interscapular region (between the shoulder blades), namely, the middle trapezius and rhomboids. The serratus anterior plays a greater role in keeping the shoulder blade against the rib cage when the arm is raised forward. The interscapular muscles are more involved in keeping the shoulder blade against the rib cage when the arm is raised to the side.

If the rotator cuff strains, in most cases you can expect that either the serratus anterior or the interscapular muscles have strained as well. Another very important muscle to check for strain along with the rotator cuff is the lower trapezius muscle. This is a muscle that plays a major role in shoulder motion and function. Once the shoulder is raised over shoulder height, the muscles of the shoulder joint play a smaller role in motion. The majority of the motion that occurs over shoulder height consists of the shoulder blade being pulled down the back by the contraction of the lower trap muscle. I have found in many cases that when there is shoulder dysfunction due to a rotator cuff strain, there is a correlative strain or weakness found with the lower trap muscle.

To see if your pain is coming from shoulder impingement from a strained rotator cuff, we'll do a range-of-motion test, some palpation, muscle testing, and flexibility testing.

Range-of-Motion Test: The first test for impingement syndrome is simply raising the arm of your affected shoulder forward as high as it can go in order to check your active range of motion. If there is a limitation and pain experienced, this is a sign that an impingement may have occurred. To confirm that the cause is not structural, such as a bone spur or bursitis, have somebody else raise your arm. This will test your passive range of motion. If your passive range of motion is full or at least substantially larger than your active range of motion, there is no structural impediment causing the shoulder region pain.

Palpation: The next test is palpation. Remember, in this test, we're trying to elicit pain in order to see which muscle is causing your pain. Try to feel for the biceps tendon. If impingement of the biceps tendon has occurred, this tendon will be thickened and prominent. It will also be painful to touch. If these symptoms are found, this is an indicator that the cause of the shoulder region pain is impingement syndrome.

Now let's palpate the infraspinatus. This muscle typically strains at the lower portion, so feel for knots and painful points along the muscle, but take extra care to notice what's happening in the lower portion. If knots or painful spots are found, this is another indicator of impingement syndrome.

Muscle Testing: Finally, we'll do some muscle testing in order to compare strength in your unaffected arm with your affected arm. You'll need someone to help you out with this one.

Place both of your arms in front of you at shoulder height. Then have your helper try to push them down. If it is easier for your helper to push the arm down on the affected side, this is an indicator of impingement syndrome.

Now raise your arms out to the side to shoulder height. Then have your helper try to push the arms down. If it is easier for your helper to push down on the affected side, this is a positive indicator of impingement syndrome.

If it is easier for your helper to push the affected arm down while doing the test with the arms in front of you, then you are weaker in flexion, and this indicates that along with the rotator cuff, the serratus anterior has strained. If it is easier to push the affected arm down while doing the test with the arms out to the sides, you are weaker in abduction. This indicates that along with the rotator cuff, the interscapular muscles have strained.

Next, we will test the rotator cuffs to see if there is a strain. To muscle test the rotator cuffs you will need someone to help you. On the unaffected side, keeping the top of your arm flush against your body, bend your elbow to 90 degrees. Your forearm will be facing forward and your hand will be thumb side up, as if you're positioning it to shake hands with someone. Have your helper place one hand on the outside of your elbow and the other on the back of the wrist. He or she will then try to push your wrist inward while you try to resist outward. Do the same test on the affected side. If the rotator cuff on the affected side is weaker, this is a positive sign that the rotator cuff has strained.

MUSCLE TESTING—SHOULDER EXTERNAL ROTATION

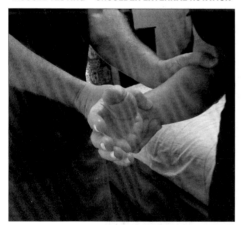

MUSCLE TESTING—SHOULDER INTERNAL ROTATION

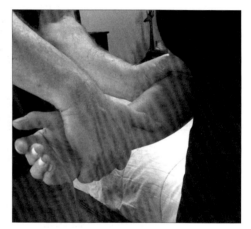

Flexibility Test: Looking at the flexibility of the rotator cuff will help determine the extent of the strain to this muscle group along with which exercises should be performed to heal. To test the flexibility of the rotator cuff, you will again need your helper. Raise your arm on the painful side out to the side up to shoulder height and bend your elbow 90 degrees, keeping your forearm and palm facing down. Your helper will stand at the elbow of your outstretched arm and place one hand at the back of your shoulder and the inside of their elbow under your elbow. The goal here is to stabilize your upper arm. With the other hand, he or she will begin to apply pressure to the top of your wrist. You will not resist this. Your helper will continue this pressure, rotating your shoulder while circling your forearm down but keeping your upper arm in place. This test should be performed slowly, and as soon as pain is elicited, the position of the shoulder rotation should be noted.

FLEXIBILITY TESTING—INTO INTERNAL ROTATION

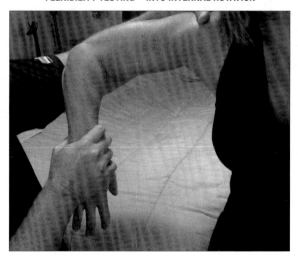

If the rotator cuff can be stretched to 90 degrees of internal rotation (moved so your fingers are pointing to the floor) without pain, then the muscle has not shortened and you will simply work to strengthen this muscle group. However, if the rotator cuff cannot be stretched to 90 degrees of internal rotation without pain, then you must first work to lengthen this muscle group before strengthening it. If a muscle is shortened and you try to strengthen it, it will simply shorten further.

The key to knowing which exercise to perform to start treating a rotator cuff strain is first determining whether the rotator cuff is at its optimal length or if it is shortened. The other key finding to determine is which of the shoulder blade stabilizing muscles have strained along with the rotator cuff. To create the right combination for your pain, you will do the following exercises only on the affected side:

1. If the rotator cuff is found to be shortened, then perform Internal Rotation of the shoulder (page 234).

2. If the rotator cuff is found to be at the optimal length, then perform External Rotation of the shoulder (page 234).

3. If the shoulder is tested and found to be weaker in flexion, then strengthen the serratus anterior by performing Protraction Punch (page 238).

4. If the shoulder is tested and found to be weaker in abduction, then strengthen the interscapular muscles (mid-traps/rhomboids) performing Lat Pulldown with Neutral Bar or Elastic Band (page 235).

The other muscles to strengthen when resolving a rotator cuff strain are the posterior deltoids, the triceps, and the lower traps on the affected side. These muscles should be strengthened regardless of the findings regarding the length of the rotator cuff and which shoulder stabilizing muscle has strained along with the rotator cuff. The exercises to perform to strengthen these muscles are:

1. Posterior Deltoids (page 237)

2. Skull Crushers (page 239)

3. Lower Trap Exercise (page 236)

PAIN IN THE BACK OF THE SHOULDER

Another fairly common location for pain at the shoulder region is the back of the shoulder. This area is anywhere between the shoulder blade and the acromion process, the top boundary of the shoulder joint. The premise for the pain in this location is the same as that for impingement syndrome. The cause is a strain of the rotator cuff. Again, let me reinforce that I am describing a rotator cuff strain, not a tear.

In this particular situation, it is actually the rotator cuff that is emitting the pain. The largest portion of the rotator cuff is a muscle called the infraspinatus. It is in the best position to perform the primary functions of the rotator cuff: namely, to maintain congruency between the head of the upper arm bone and the shoulder joint as well as to depress the head of the upper arm bone to prevent it impacting the acromion process during shoulder motion. This muscle spans a large portion of the shoulder blade. If it strains, it can cause pain to be emitted anywhere within the boundary of the muscle. For most people, the pain is experienced at the top of the muscle where it joins with its tendon and begins to attach to the head of the upper arm bone. If you feel for the back of the acromion process and then feel just below this, this is the typical location where a strained infraspinatus will emit pain. However, some people with this strain complain of pain all the way down at the bottom of the shoulder blade.

Resolving pain at the back of the shoulder due to a rotator cuff strain is the same as with an impingement of the biceps. All the associated muscles that may have strained along with the rotator cuff must be identified, and a complete strengthening program must be developed to maximize the strength of all relevant muscles.

To see if the pain at the posterior shoulder is coming from a strained rotator cuff, we'll do some palpation, muscle testing, and a flexibility test.

Palpation: The first test is palpation. Remember, in this test, we're trying to elicit pain in order to see which muscle is causing your pain. Try to feel for the infraspinatus muscle. Feel all the way from its attachment, which can be felt just below the back of the acromion process all the way down to the lowest portion of the shoulder blade. I have found that straining of the infraspinatus is most common near the bottom of the shoulder blade. If knots are found, it will be painful to touch. If these symptoms are found, this is an indicator that the cause of the posterior shoulder region pain is a strained rotator cuff.

Muscle Testing: Next, we'll do some muscle testing in order to compare strength in your unaffected arm with your affected arm. You'll need someone to help you out with this one.

Place both of your arms in front of you at shoulder height. Then have your helper try to push them down. If it is easier for your helper to push the arm down on the affected side, this is an indicator of a strained rotator cuff.

Now raise your arms out to the side to shoulder height. Then have your helper try to push the arms down. If it is easier for your helper to push down on the affected side, this is a positive indicator of a strained rotator cuff.

If it is easier for your helper to push the affected arm down while doing the test with the arms in front of you, then you are weaker in flexion, and this indicates that along with the rotator cuff, the serratus anterior has strained. If it is easier to push the affected arm down while doing the test with the arms out to the sides, you are weaker in abduction, and this indicates that along with the rotator cuff the interscapular muscles have strained.

Next, we will test the rotator cuffs to see if there is a strain. To muscle test the rotator cuffs you will need someone to help you. On the unaffected side, keeping the top of your arm flush against your body, bend your elbow to 90 degrees. Your forearm will be facing forward and your hand will be thumb side up, as if you're positioning it to shake hands with someone. Have your helper place one hand on the outside of your elbow and the other on the back of the wrist. He or she will then try to push your wrist inward while you try to resist outward. Do the same test on the affected side. If the rotator cuff on the affected side is weaker, this is a positive sign that the rotator cuff has strained.

MUSCLE TESTING—SHOULDER EXTERNAL ROTATION

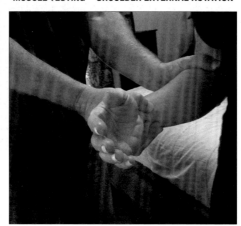

Flexibility Test: Looking at the flexibility of the rotator cuff will help determine the extent of the strain to this muscle group along with which exercises should be performed to heal. To test the flexibility of the rotator cuff, you will again need your helper. Raise your arm on the painful side out to the side up to shoulder height and bend your elbow 90 degrees, keeping your forearm and palm facing down. Your helper will stand at the elbow of your outstretched arm and place one hand at the back of your shoulder and the inside of his or her elbow under your elbow. The goal here is to stabilize your upper arm. With the other hand, he or she will begin to apply pressure to the top of your wrist. You will not resist this. Your helper will continue this pressure, rotating your shoulder while circling your forearm down but keeping your upper arm in place. This test should be performed slowly, and as soon as pain is elicited, the position of the shoulder rotation should be noted.

FLEXIBILITY TESTING—INTO INTERNAL ROTATION

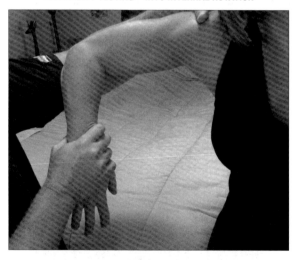

If the rotator cuff can be stretched to 90 degrees of internal rotation (moved so your fingers are pointing to the floor) without pain, then the muscle has not shortened and you will simply work to strengthen this muscle group. However, if the rotator cuff cannot be stretched to 90 degrees of internal rotation without pain, then you must first work to lengthen this muscle group before strengthening it. If a muscle is shortened, and you try to strengthen it, it will simply shorten further.

The key to knowing which exercise to perform to start treating a rotator cuff strain is first determining whether the rotator cuff is at its optimal length or if it is shortened. The other key finding to determine is which of the shoulder blade stabilizing muscles have strained along with the rotator cuff, to create the right combination for your pain. You will do the following exercises only on the affected side:

1. If the rotator cuff is found to be shortened, then perform Internal Rotation of the shoulder (page 234).

2. If the rotator cuff is found to be at the optimal length, then perform External Rotation of the shoulder (page 234).

3. If the shoulder is tested and found to be weaker in flexion, then strengthen the serratus anterior by performing Protraction Punch (page 238).

4. If the shoulder is tested and found to be weaker in abduction, then strengthen the interscapular muscles (mid-traps/rhomboids) performing Lat Pulldown with Neutral Bar or Elastic Band (page 235).

The other muscles to strengthen when resolving a rotator cuff strain are the posterior deltoids, the triceps, and the lower traps on the affected side. These muscles should be strengthened regardless of the findings regarding the length of the rotator cuff and which shoulder stabilizing muscle has strained along with the rotator cuff. The exercises to perform to strengthen these muscles are:

1. Posterior Deltoids (page 237)

2. Skull Crushers (page 239)

3. Lower Trap Exercise (page 236)

PAIN AT THE SIDE OF THE SHOULDER AND THE UPPER ARM

MUSCLES OF THE UPPER ARM—LATERAL VIEW

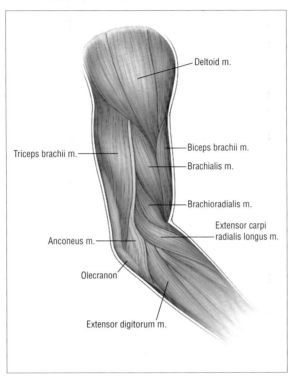

As noted in the section above, a strain of the rotator cuff can lead to impingement syndrome, which will typically create pain at the front of the shoulder. There are, however, many people who experience pain at the side of the shoulder and the upper arm. In almost every case I've seen where the pain is in these places, the tissue emitting the pain is the brachialis muscle, which is an elbow flexor, meaning that it bends the elbow. It attaches high on the outside of the upper arm bone.

Why does a muscle associated with the elbow affect the shoulder? Think about the two ways you can raise your hand to eye height. Either you can keep your elbow straight, raising your arm from the shoulder, or you simply bend your elbow to raise your hand. A strain of the rotator cuff and other supporting muscles in the shoulder leads to overuse of the latter movement (bending through the elbow). This causes the brachialis to overwork, strain, and break down, creating pain where it attaches at the upper arm.

The tests for confirming that a strained brachialis is the cause of pain at the side portion of the shoulder and upper arm are the same as those for confirming that a strain of the rotator cuff and other supporting muscles has occurred. Test to see if there is a rotator cuff muscle strain and whether there is a shoulder blade stabilizing muscle that has strained.

Palpation: The first test is palpation. Remember, in this test, we're trying to elicit pain in order to see which muscle is causing your pain. Try to feel for the brachialis muscle. If the muscle has strained, it will be thickened and prominent. It will also be painful to touch. If these symptoms are found, this is an indicator that the cause of the lateral shoulder and upper arm pain is a brachialis strain.

Now let's palpate the infraspinatus. This muscle typically strains at the lower portion, so feel for knots and painful points along the muscle but take extra care to notice what's happening in the lower portion. If knots or painful spots are found, this is another indicator of a brachialis strain.

Muscle Testing: Next, we'll do some muscle testing in order to compare strength in your unaffected arm with your affected arm. You'll need someone to help you out with this one.

Place both of your arms in front of you at shoulder height. Then have your helper try to push them down. If it is easier for your helper to push the arm down on the affected side, this is an indicator of a brachialis strain.

Now try the test again with both arms. This time, raise your arms out to the side to shoulder height. Then have your helper try to push the arms down. If it is easier for your helper to push down on the affected side, this is a positive indicator of a brachialis strain.

If it is easier for your helper to push the affected arm down while doing the test with the arms in front of you, then you are weaker in flexion, and this indicates that along with the rotator cuff, the serratus anterior has strained. If it is easier to push the affected arm down while doing the test with the arms out to the sides, you are weaker in abduction, and this indicates that along with the rotator cuff the interscapular muscles have strained.

Next, we will test the rotator cuffs to see if there is a strain. To muscle test the rotator cuffs you will need someone to help you. On the unaffected side, keeping the top of your arm flush against your body, bend your elbow to 90 degrees. Your forearm will be facing forward and your hand will be thumb side up, as if you're positioning it to shake hands with someone. Next, have your helper place one hand on the outside of your elbow and the other on the back of the wrist. He or she will then try to push your wrist inward while you try to resist outward. Then do the same test on the affected side. If the rotator cuff on the affected side is weaker, this is a positive sign that the rotator cuff has strained.

MUSCLE TESTING—SHOULDER EXTERNAL ROTATION

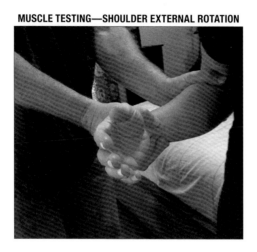

Flexibility Test: Looking at the flexibility of the rotator cuff will help determine the extent of the strain to this muscle group along with which exercises should be performed to heal. To test the flexibility of the rotator cuff, you will again need your helper. Raise your arm on the painful side out to the side up to shoulder height and bend your elbow 90 degrees, keeping your forearm and palm facing down. Your helper will stand at the elbow of your outstretched arm and place one hand at the back of your shoulder and the inside of his or her elbow under your elbow. The goal here is to stabilize your upper arm. With the other hand, he or she will begin to apply pressure to the top of your wrist. You will not resist this. Your helper will continue this pressure, rotating your shoulder while circling your forearm down but keeping your upper arm in place. This test should be performed slowly, and as soon as pain is elicited, the position of the shoulder rotation should be noted.

FLEXIBILITY TESTING—INTO INTERNAL ROTATION

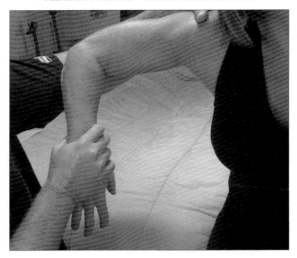

If the rotator cuff can be stretched to 90 degrees of internal rotation (moved so your fingers are pointing to the floor) without pain, then the muscle has not shortened and you will simply work to strengthen this muscle group. However, if the rotator cuff cannot be stretched to 90 degrees of internal rotation without pain, then you must first work to lengthen this muscle group before strengthening it. If a muscle is shortened, and you try to strengthen it, it will simply shorten further.

The key to knowing which exercise to perform to start treating a rotator cuff strain is first determining whether the rotator cuff is at its optimal length or if it is shortened. The other key finding to determine is which of the shoulder blade stabilizing muscles have strained along with the rotator cuff, to create the right combination for your pain. You will do the following exercises only on the affected side:

1. If the rotator cuff is found to be shortened, then perform Internal Rotation of the shoulder (page 234).

2. If the rotator cuff is found to be at the optimal length, then perform External Rotation of the shoulder (page 234).

3. If the shoulder is tested and found to be weaker in flexion, then strengthen the serratus anterior by performing Protraction Punch (page 238).

4. If the shoulder is tested and found to be weaker in abduction, then strengthen the interscapular muscles (mid-traps/rhomboids) by performing Lat Pulldown with Neutral Bar or Elastic Band (page 235).

The other muscles to strengthen when resolving a rotator cuff strain are the posterior deltoids, the triceps, and the lower traps on the affected side. These muscles should be strengthened regardless of the findings regarding the length of the rotator cuff and which shoulder stabilizing muscle has strained along with the rotator cuff. The exercises to perform to strengthen these muscles are:

1. Posterior Deltoids (page 237)

2. Skull Crushers (page 239)

3. Lower Trap Exercise (page 236)

PAIN UNDER THE ARM OR IN THE ARMPIT

As I have discussed, there is a strong relationship between the shoulder blade stabilizing muscles and the rotator cuff. Many of these lead to a strain of some other muscle; however, in some cases the shoulder blade stabilizing muscles themselves can create pain. A strain of the serratus anterior, which attaches from the underside of the shoulder blade to eight ribs, can actually mimic the symptoms of a heart attack. If this muscle spasms, it can limit the ability of the rib cage to expand and contract, causing shortness of breath and pain at the side of the rib cage. Patients can also describe themselves as having pain under the arm or in the armpit.

A strain of interscapular muscles, which sit between the inside border of the shoulder blade and the spine, has often been misdiagnosed as a compression fracture of the spine or a herniated disc.

To see if the pain you are experiencing at the mid-back or under the arm/armpit is coming from a strained shoulder blade stabilizing muscle, we'll do some palpation, muscle testing, and a flexibility test.

Palpation: The first test is palpation. Remember, in this test, we're trying to elicit pain in order to see which muscle is causing your pain. Try to feel for the interscapular muscles or the serratus anterior. If strained, the muscles will be thickened and prominent. They will also be painful to touch. If these symptoms are found, this is an indicator that the cause of the shoulder region pain is a strain of the interscapular muscles or serratus anterior.

Now let's palpate the infraspinatus. This muscle typically strains at the lower portion, so feel for knots and painful points along the muscle, but take extra care to notice what's happening in the lower portion. If knots or painful spots are found, this is another indicator of a strain of the interscapular muscles or serratus anterior.

Muscle Testing: Next, we'll do some muscle testing in order to compare strength in your unaffected arm with your affected arm. You'll need someone to help you out with this one.

Place both of your arms in front of you at shoulder height. Then have your helper try to push them down. If it is easier for your helper to push the arm down on the affected side, this is an indicator of a strain of the interscapular muscles or serratus anterior.

Now try the test again with both arms. This time, raise your arms out to the side to shoulder height. Then have your helper try to push the arms down. If it is easier for your helper to push down on the affected side, this is a positive indicator of a strain of the interscapular muscles or serratus anterior.

If it is easier for your helper to push the affected arm down while doing the test with the arms in front of you, then you are weaker in flexion, and this indicates that along with the rotator cuff, the serratus anterior has strained. If it is easier to push the affected arm down while doing the test with the arms out to the sides, you are weaker in abduction, and this indicates that along with the rotator cuff, the interscapular muscles have strained.

Next, we will test the rotator cuffs to see if there is a strain. To muscle test the rotator cuffs you will need someone to help you. On the unaffected side, keeping the top of your arm flush against your body, bend your elbow to 90 degrees. Your forearm will be facing forward and your hand will be thumb side up, as if you're positioning it to shake hands with someone. Next, have your helper place one hand on the outside of your elbow and the other on the back of the wrist. He or she will then try to push your wrist inward while you try to resist outward. Then do the same test on the affected side. If the rotator cuff on the affected side is weaker, this is a positive sign that the rotator cuff has strained.

MUSCLE TESTING—SHOULDER EXTERNAL ROTATION

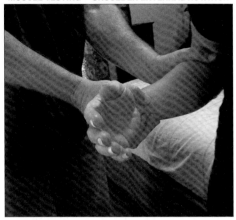

Flexibility Test: Looking at the flexibility of the rotator cuff will help determine the extent of the strain to this muscle group along with which exercises should be performed to heal. To test the flexibility of the rotator cuff, you will again need your helper. Raise your arm on the painful side out to the side up to shoulder height and bend your elbow 90 degrees, keeping your forearm and palm facing down. Your helper will stand at the elbow of your outstretched arm and place one hand at the back of your shoulder and the inside of his or her elbow under your elbow. The goal here is to stabilize your upper arm. With the other hand, he or she will begin to apply pressure to the top of your wrist. You will not resist this. Your helper will continue this pressure, rotating your shoulder while circling your forearm down but keeping your upper arm in place. This test should be performed slowly, and as soon as pain is elicited, the position of the shoulder rotation should be noted.

FLEXIBILITY TESTING—INTO INTERNAL ROTATION

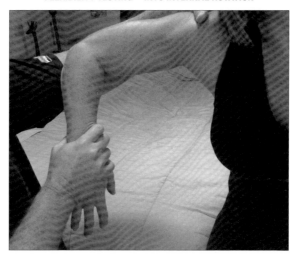

If the rotator cuff can be stretched to 90 degrees of internal rotation (moved so your fingers are pointing to the floor) without pain, then the muscle has not shortened and you will simply work to strengthen this muscle group. However, if the rotator cuff cannot be stretched to 90 degrees of internal rotation without pain, then you must first work to lengthen this muscle group before strengthening it. If a muscle is shortened, and you try to strengthen it, it will simply shorten further.

The key to knowing which exercise to perform to start treating a rotator cuff strain is first determining whether the rotator cuff is at its optimal length or if it is shortened. The other key finding to determine is which of the shoulder blade stabilizing muscles have strained along with the rotator cuff, to create the right combination for your pain. You will do the following exercises only on the affected side:

1. If the rotator cuff is found to be shortened, then perform Internal Rotation of the shoulder (page 234).

2. If the rotator cuff is found to be at the optimal length, then perform External Rotation of the shoulder (page 234).

3. If the shoulder is tested and found to be weaker in flexion, then strengthen the serratus anterior by performing Protraction Punch (page 234).

4. If the shoulder is tested and found to be weaker in abduction, then strengthen the interscapular muscles (mid-traps/rhomboids) performing Lat Pulldown with Neutral Bar or Elastic Band (page 235).

The other muscles to strengthen when resolving a rotator cuff strain are the posterior deltoids, the triceps, and the lower traps on the affected side. These muscles should be strengthened regardless of the findings regarding the length of the rotator cuff and which shoulder stabilizing muscle has strained along with the rotator cuff. The exercises to perform to strengthen these muscles are:

1. Posterior Deltoids (page 237)

2. Skull Crushers (page 239)

3. Lower Trap Exercise (page 236)

CHAPTER 11

THE **HIP** AND **GROIN**

BONY ANATOMY OF THE HIP JOINT

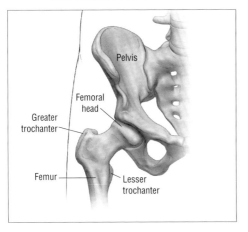

Pelvis

Femoral head

Greater trochanter

Femur

Lesser trochanter

ARTHRITIS OF THE HIP JOINT

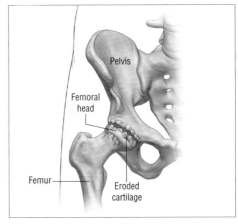

Pelvis

Femoral head

Femur

Eroded cartilage

MUSCLES OF THE THIGH—ANTERIOR VIEW

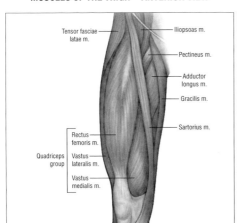

Tensor fasciae latae m.

Iliopsoas m.

Pectineus m.

Adductor longus m.

Gracilis m.

Sartorius m.

Rectus femoris m.

Quadriceps group

Vastus lateralis m.

Vastus medialis m.

MUSCLES OF THE GLUTEAL REGION

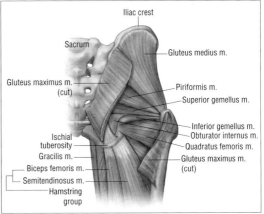

Iliac crest

Sacrum

Gluteus medius m.

Gluteus maximus m. (cut)

Piriformis m.

Superior gemellus m.

Inferior gemellus m.

Obturator internus m.

Quadratus femoris m.

Gluteus maximus m. (cut)

Ischial tuberosity

Gracilis m.

Biceps femoris m.

Semitendinosus m.

Hamstring group

In this chapter you will find a description of the muscle groups possibly involved in creating pain in your hip and groin regions, along with clinical tests to confirm which muscle is emitting the pain. Once you have determined where the pain is coming from, please go to the Appendix to learn the muscle-strengthening and stretching exercises that will help resolve your pain.

The hip region pertains to the area around the hip joint. This is the location where the head of the femur (thigh bone) attaches into the pelvis. Oddly, most people aren't sure where the hip joint is located. When asked to identify the hip joint, most people point to the top of the pelvis. I think the concept comes from this idea: when somebody says put your hands on your hips, most people will put their hands on the top or rim of the pelvis. The actual hip joint is lower. Simply move your hands down from the rim of the pelvis to the side of your outer thigh until you feel a bony prominence, which represents the head of the thigh bone entering the pelvis. This chapter will present how to differentiate between the different muscle imbalances that can cause pain at the hip.

I will also cover groin region pain in this chapter, because the hip and the groin are so integrally related—and often groin pain will be blamed on a hip dysfunction. However, there are muscles in the groin region that can strain and emit pain.

HIP PAIN

Possibility 1: Strained Gluteus Medius

A strained gluteus medius (glute med) is by far the number one muscular cause of hip region pain. The gluteus medius, which sits directly above the hip joint and attaches from the top of the pelvis to the hip joint, plays a pivotal role in supporting you, especially when standing on one leg, as in the case of walking. The glute med keeps the pelvis level when standing on one leg so balance is maintained. If the glute med is weak and you are standing on the affected side, the pelvis on the opposite side will begin to drop toward the floor. This shifts your center of mass from over the leg you are standing on to the midline of the body.

The reason that the glute med might strain is that it does not have enough strength to perform the functional activities you are trying to perform. It might also be related to other muscles in the leg being weak, and therefore the glute med strains in compensating for the weakness of the other muscles.

If the glute med has strained, it can elicit pain anywhere along the length of the muscle. This means that pain can be experienced close to the glute med's attachment to the head of the femur at the hip joint.

To determine whether or not a strained glute med is the cause of your pain, we'll do palpation, muscle testing, and posture analysis.

Palpation: The first test to determine whether the cause of the hip region pain is a gluteus medius strain is palpation. Feel for the top of the pelvis, and then begin to feel down, moving toward the hip joint, pressing and feeling for knots in the gluteus medius muscle. If pain or knots are identified, this is the first indicator that the cause of the hip region pain is a gluteus medius strain.

Muscle Testing: To perform this test, you'll need the help of someone else. First, lie down on a firm surface on your side. Raise your top leg a few inches, so it runs parallel to the floor. Make sure to keep it in line with your torso, not drifting forward or backward. Have your helper place one hand on your pelvis just above the hip joint and the other on your ankle. Try to push up at the ankle while the person tries to stop you. Then turn over and try the same test with the other leg. If the glute med is weaker on the same side that you are having the hip pain, this is an indication that the strained glute med is the cause of your pain. There should be a noticeable difference in muscle strength between the unaffected and affected sides.

MUSCLE TESTING—GLUTEUS MEDIUS

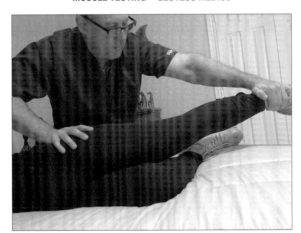

Posture Analysis: The next thing you'll want to do is look at your posture. Stand in front of a mirror that can provide a full view of you from the front. Place your hands on the rim of your pelvis (most people consider this their hips) and see if one hand is higher than the other. If the glute med has strained, the pelvis on the opposite side will drop. Eventually, this will cause the lower back muscles to shorten in order to compensate, and those muscles will pull that same side up, causing it to be elevated. If the hip opposite your painful hip is elevated, this is another indicator that the cause of the hip region pain is a gluteus medius strain.

STANDING POSTURE—NORMAL   **STANDING POSTURE—HIP HIKED**

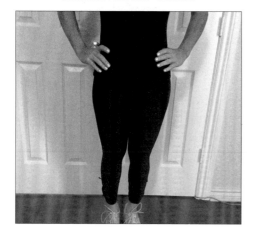
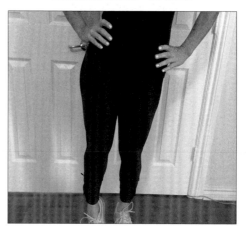

Finally, you can look at posture while walking. You will need someone to help you with this. Have the person stand behind you as you walk slowly away from him or her. As you are walking, the person should look to see if either of your hips dips down when taking a step through. He or she should watch the hip of the leg that is swinging forward just as the leg is lifted. Since the glute med plays an important role in stabilizing the pelvis, if it is weakened, the hip opposite the strained glute med will dip as you walk.

WALKING POSTURE—NORMAL

WALKING POSTURE—HIP DROP

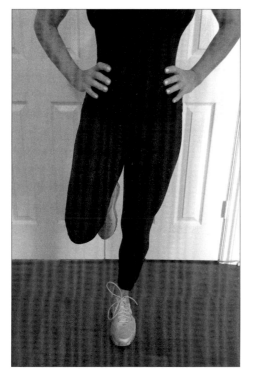
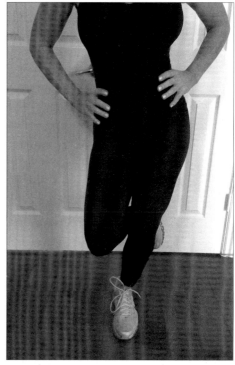

If the hips stay even when the painful hip is in motion (when the unaffected leg is stood on), but the non-painful hip dips when the unaffected leg is in motion (when the painful leg is stood on), this is an indication that the strained glute med is causing your pain.

WALKING POSTURE—NORMAL   **WALKING POSTURE—SIDEBENT**

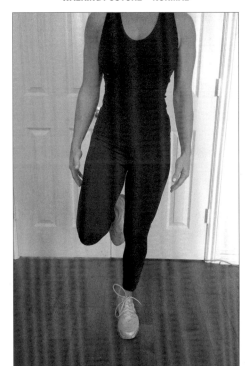 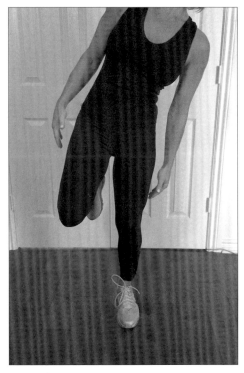

Another possible compensation that occurs when you have a strained glute med is that you bend to the side of the affected leg whenever that leg is stood on. By bending to the side of the injured leg, your body weight moves over the leg, which prevents the need for support of the weight by the strained glute med. If your helper sees this when watching you walk, this is another indication that a strained glute med is your problem.

Sidebending is common among the older population or in people who have had joint replacements. Even though most of these people are told that sidebending is due to old age or their hip replacement, this movement is almost exclusively associated with a weak gluteus medius muscle. Unfortunately, this sidebending can also lead to instability and falls, which is why I'm bringing it up. Please know that this is completely treatable.

If the gluteus medius is the muscle that has strained and is causing pain at the hip region, the muscles to strengthen are the gluteus medius muscle, the gluteus maximus, and the hamstrings. The exercises to be performed are:

1. Hip Abduction in sidelying or with a cable system (page 241)

2. Hamstring Curl (page 240)

3. Straight Leg Deadlifts (page 246)

Possibility 2: Strained ITB

The other possible muscular cause of hip pain is a strained ITB (iliotibial) band, which is often caused by a strained glute med.

The ITB band is a long thick band of connective tissue that runs from the outer top portion of the pelvis to the outside of the knee. It is tightened and controlled by a small muscle called the tensor fasciae latae. This grouping works with the gluteus medius muscle to create pelvic support. If the glute med strains, this can cause the tensor fasciae latae to overwork to compensate, which leads it to strain. In turn, this causes altered tension on the ITB band, which makes it thicken and become painful.

The pain from this strain is normally felt just below the hip joint or along the outside part of the thigh. The key to identifying the ITB band as the cause of this pain versus another possibility like sciatica is the fact that this pain will go no farther than the knee.

I said above that the strained ITB band is *likely* due to a strained glute med; however, I would like to point out that the ITB band does pass across the hip joint during some motions of the hip, and it is possible for the ITB band to become irritated and painful from this. But these are rare cases. If your hip hurts and you feel a snapping sensation when you move it, this could be the cause. Some people describe the feeling as the hip dislocating—even though this is not possible. Because this is so rare, I will not cover it in this book.

To find out if a strained ITB band is the cause of your hip pain, you will do palpation, flexibility testing, muscle testing, and posture analysis.

Palpation: The first test to identify a strained ITB band is palpation. Remember, our goal here is to find the muscle that is strained by eliciting pain through pressure. Press along the ITB band from its attachment at the pelvis, down the outside of the thigh, and on to its attachment to the lower leg bone at the fibular head. If you feel pain anywhere along the band, this is the first indicator that the lateral hip region pain is coming from a strained ITB band.

Flexibility Testing: A strained ITB band will prevent external rotation of the hip from occurring. In this test, we will test both legs in order to compare flexibility. Simply place the ankle of one leg on the knee of the other leg when sitting. First, try to put the ankle of your unaffected leg on the knee of your leg with hip pain. Then switch. If it is more difficult to perform this action with the affected leg, it is another indicator that the cause of your hip pain is a strained ITB band. If the ITB band has strained significantly enough, you may be unable to do this action at all. The action might also create pain, which reinforces the strained ITB band as the cause of the pain.

FLEXIBILITY TESTING—ITB

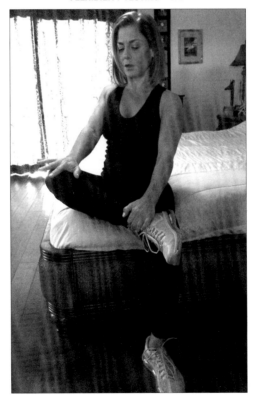

Muscle Testing: The muscle test and the posture analysis described below are used to confirm the existence of a strained glute med, which could lead to a strained ITB band. To perform the muscle test, you'll need the help of someone else.

MUSCLE TESTING—GLUTEUS MEDIUS

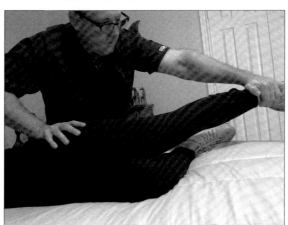

Lie down on a firm surface on your side. Raise your top leg a few inches, so it runs parallel to the floor. Make sure to keep it in line with your torso, not drifting forward or backward. Have your helper place one hand on your pelvis just above the hip joint and the other on your ankle. Try to push up at the ankle while the person tries to stop you. Then turn over and try the same test with the other leg. If the leg with the hip pain is found to be weaker, this is another indication that the cause of your hip pain is an ITB band strain caused by a strained glute med.

Posture Analysis: To do the posture analysis, stand in front of a mirror that can provide a full view of you from the front. Place your hands on the rim of your pelvis (most people consider this their hips) and see if one hand is higher than the other. If the glute med has strained, the pelvis on the opposite side will drop. Eventually, this will cause the lower back muscles to shorten in order to compensate, and those muscles will pull that same side up, causing it to be elevated. If your hip opposite your painful hip is elevated, this is another indicator that the ITB band may be strained as a result of a glute med strain.

STANDING POSTURE—NORMAL

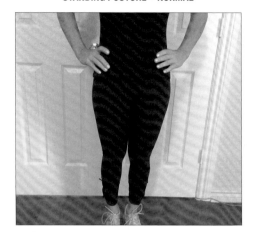

STANDING POSTURE—HIP HIKED

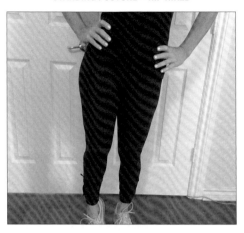

Finally, you can look at posture while walking. You will need someone to help you with this. Have the person stand behind you as you walk slowly away from him or her. As you are walking, the person should look to see if either of your hips dips down when taking a step through. He or she should watch the hip of the leg that is swinging forward just as the leg is lifted. Since the glute med plays an important role in stabilizing the pelvis, if it is weakened, the hip will dip as you walk.

WALKING POSTURE—NORMAL

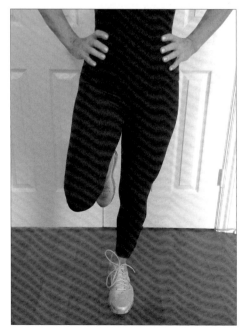

WALKING POSTURE—HIP DROP

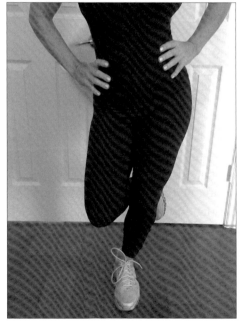

If the hips stay even when the affected leg is in motion (when the unaffected leg is stood on), but the hip dips when the unaffected leg is in motion (when the painful leg is stood on), this is an indication of a strained glute med, which could have led to an ITB band strain.

WALKING POSTURE—NORMAL **WALKING POSTURE—SIDEBENT**

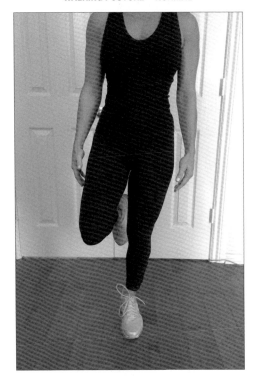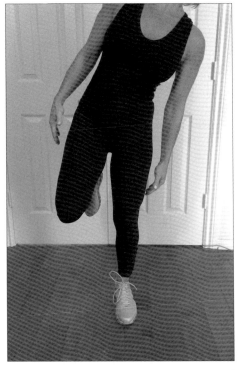

Another possible compensation that occurs when you have a strained glute med is that you bend to the side of the affected leg whenever that leg is stood on. By bending to the side of the injured leg, your body weight moves over the leg, which prevents the need for support of the weight by the strained glute med. If your helper sees this when watching you walk, this is another indication that a strained glute med could have led to a strained ITB band.

Sidebending is common among the older population or in people who have had joint replacements. Even though most of these people are told that sidebending is due to old age or their hip replacement, this movement is almost exclusively associated with a weak gluteus medius muscle. Unfortunately, this sidebending can also lead to instability and falls, which is why I'm bringing it up. Please know that this is completely treatable.

If the cause of your hip region pain is a strained ITB, the muscles that need to be strengthened are the gluteus medius, gluteus maximus, and the quads; the ITB band also needs to be stretched. The exercises that should be performed are:

1. Hip Abduction in sidelying or with a cable system (page 241)
2. Hip Extension with a resistance band or cable system (page 242)
3. Knee Extension (page 242)
4. ITB Stretch (page 248)

Once the ITB band has been lengthened to its optimal length, do the following:

1. Hip Extension with a resistance band or cable system (page 242)
2. Straight Leg Deadlifts (page 246)
3. Hamstring Curl (page 240)

Possibility 3: Strained Piriformis

A strained piriformis muscle is the final possibility for creating pain in the hip region. A strain in the piriformis is interesting because it can cause pain anywhere between its attachment to the sacral spine in the gluteal region to its attachment to the hip joint.

The piriformis muscle will typically strain if the gluteus medius muscle has strained first. The glute med and the piriformis muscle both act as pelvic stabilizing muscles. These muscles help to stabilize the pelvis so muscles like the quads and hamstrings, which are responsible for creating locomotion, can pull on the pelvis to create force and perform this functional role. If the gluteus medius muscle strains and emits pain, it will create pain just above the hip joint. If the piriformis strains and emits pain, that strain can reach to the gluteal region.

To find out if your hip pain is coming from a strained piriformis—along with which glute med led to the piriformis strain—you will do posture analysis, a single leg standing test, a muscle test, and some palpation.

Posture Analysis: The first test we can look at is hip height. Stand in front of a mirror that can provide a full view of you from the front. Place your hands on the rim of your pelvis (most people consider this their hips) and see if one hand is higher than the other. If the hip is higher on the same side as your pain, this indicates that the glute med on the opposite side of your body is strained. If the hip is higher on the opposite side of your body from the pain, this indicates that the glute med on the same side as the pain is strained.

Single Leg Standing Test: The next test to look at is the single leg standing test. Try to stand on one leg, and then try to stand on the other. If one leg is more difficult to stand on, this indicates a strained glute med. Note if the strain is on the same side as your hip pain or on the opposite side.

Muscle Testing: Another way to confirm a diagnosis of a strained glute med is to test the strength of your glute meds. To perform this test, you'll need the help of someone else. First, lie down on a firm surface on your side. Raise your top leg a few inches, so it runs parallel to the floor. Make sure to keep it in line with your torso, not drifting forward or backward. Have your helper place one hand on your pelvis just above the hip joint and the other on your ankle. Try to push up at the ankle while the person tries to stop you. Then turn over and try the same test with the other leg. If the glute med is weaker on the side that you are having the hip pain, this indicates that the strained glute med is on the same side as your pain. If the glute med on the opposite side of your body is weaker, this is an indication of strain on the opposite side.

Palpation: Finally, we can do some palpation. Feel for the piriformis muscle where the pain is being experienced. See if you can find knots in the muscle and if you increase the pain in the hip region. This will indicate if the piriformis is the cause of your hip pain. Now feel for the glute med on both sides. See if you can find knots in this muscle or if pressing on it causes pain. The side where there are knots and pain is the side with the strained glute med that led to the strained piriformis.

The key to treating hip region pain is to strengthen the glute meds, gluteus maximus, and hamstrings and to stretch the piriformis muscle. While it may be obvious why we need to strengthen the glute med, we should work on the gluteus maximus and hamstrings because they are also integrally involved in support when standing on a single leg. They are both hip extensors, which help you stand upright. When you are standing upright optimally, the skeletal structure supports most of the body. This means muscles have to work less. In working less, more energy can go toward the glute meds to help create the force necessary to sustain balance when single leg standing.

As a general rule, I have found that there is no such thing as too much strength when it comes to the glute meds. So even if the gluteal region pain is created by one or the other glute med straining, I would suggest strengthening both glute meds. Start by strengthening only the weakened glute med first with Hip Abduction. Once the pain is resolved, begin to strengthen the glute med on the opposite side to achieve maximal strength of the glute meds. Other than the Hip Abduction exercise, you will perform all the following exercises only on the affected side:

1. Hip Abduction (page 241)

2. Hamstring Curl (page 240)

3. Hip Extension (page 242)

4. Straight Leg Deadlifts (page 246)

5. Piriformis Stretch (page 249)

GROIN PAIN

Remember that pain in the groin region is typically a red flag for the medical establishment that there is some type of dysfunction at the hip joint. They rarely recognize that there are tissues in the groin region that can also create pain. The ability to differentiate which tissues are emitting the pain can prevent you from getting an unnecessary hip surgery. Remember the difference between a referred pain versus point-tender pain when trying to evaluate the cause of pain in this region. The balance of the tests for each potential muscular cause will help to clarify the cause.

Possibility 1: Strained Gracilis

A strained gracilis will often cause pain in the groin region. The gracilis muscle runs down the inner thigh with attachments to the pelvis and to the knee joint at the pes anserinus. This muscle is responsible for helping create movement in the hip, and it can easily strain following a glute med strain. A glute med strain weakens the force being created for abduction (the motion moving away from the midline of the body). This causes the gracilis, which is an adductor (pulling the leg toward the midline of the body), to shorten. Once shortened, the gracilis loses its ability to create force and strains, creating pain at the groin region. Once shortened, the gracilis is also susceptible to being overstretched if the legs are separated quickly or with a large motion. This can also lead to a gracilis strain emitting pain at the groin region.

To test whether or not a strained gracilis is the cause of your groin pain, we'll do palpation, muscle testing, and posture analysis.

Palpation: The first test to perform is palpation. Remember, the goal of palpation is to elicit pain in order to see which muscle is causing your problem. Simply feel along the gracilis muscle from its attachment from the pelvis down to the knee. See if you can find areas of pain and/or knots. If so, this is the first indicator that the cause of the groin region pain is a gracilis strain.

Muscle Testing: The next test is muscle testing of the gluteus medius and gracilis. To perform these tests, you'll need the help of someone else.

MUSCLE TESTING—GLUTEUS MEDIUS

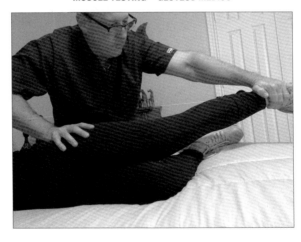

First, we'll test the glute med. Lie down on a firm surface on your side. Raise your top leg a few inches, so it runs parallel to the ground. Make sure to keep it in line with your torso, not drifting forward or backward. Have your helper place one hand on your pelvis just above the hip joint and the other on your ankle. Try to push up at the ankle while the person tries to stop you. Then turn over and try the same test with the other leg. If the leg with the groin pain is found to be weaker, this is another indication that the cause of your groin pain is a gracilis strain.

The next test is a muscle test of the gracilis muscle. You will need someone to help you perform this test. Lie down on a flat surface. Have your helper place one hand on the inside of your thigh just above the knee and one hand on the inside of the other ankle. He or she will try to stabilize the leg with the hand on the thigh while trying to pull the ankle away from the midline. You will try to resist the pressure being applied at your ankle.

MUSCLE TESTING—GRACILIS

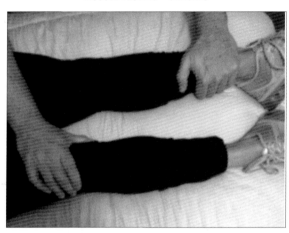

First, test the unaffected leg, pulling this ankle. Then test the affected leg. Make sure that when you are performing this test the knee of the leg being tested is straight. If you are better able to resist the force of the ankle being pulled on the unaffected leg—and less able to resist on the affected leg—this is another indicator that the groin pain is the result of a strained gracilis. If the gracilis has strained significantly enough, this test will create pain at the groin.

Posture Analysis: The posture analysis tests aim to identify a strained gluteus medius muscle in order to corroborate the diagnosis of a strained gracilis muscle causing the groin pain.

Stand in front of a mirror that can provide a full view of you from the front. Place your hands on the rim of your pelvis (most people consider this their hips) and see if one hand is higher than the other. If the glute med has strained, the pelvis on the opposite side will drop. Eventually, this will cause the lower back muscles to shorten in order to compensate, and those muscles will pull that same side up, causing it to be elevated. If the hip opposite your painful groin is elevated, this is another indicator that the cause of the groin pain is gracilis strain caused by a strained glute med.

STANDING POSTURE—NORMAL

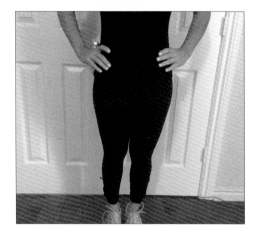

STANDING POSTURE—HIP HIKED

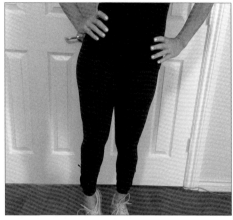

Finally, you can look at posture while walking. You will need someone to help you with this. Have the person stand behind you as you walk slowly away from him or her. As you are walking, the person should look to see if either of your hips dips down when taking a step through. He or she should watch the hip of the leg that is swinging forward just as the leg is lifted. Since the glute med plays an important role in stabilizing the pelvis, if it is weakened, the hip will dip as you walk.

STANDING POSTURE—NORMAL

STANDING POSTURE—HIP DROP

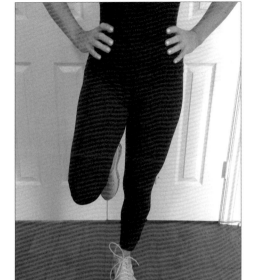
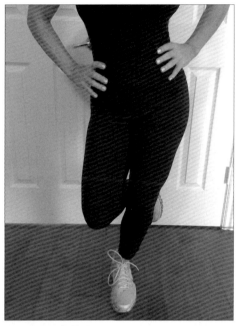

If the hips stay even when the affected leg is in motion (when the unaffected leg is stood on), but the hip dips when the unaffected leg is in motion (when the painful leg is stood on), this is an indication of a strained glute med, which could have led to a gracilis strain.

STANDING POSTURE—NORMAL **STANDING POSTURE—SIDEBENT**

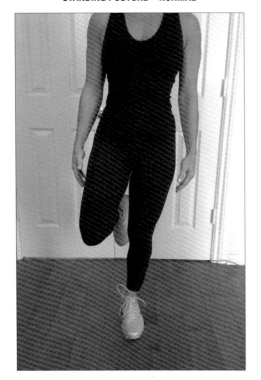 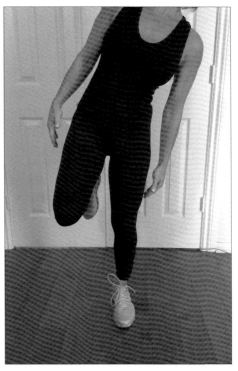

Another possible compensation that occurs when you have a strained glute med is that you bend to the side of the affected leg whenever that leg is stood on. By bending to the side of the injured leg, your body weight moves over the leg, which prevents the need for support of the weight by the strained glute med. If your helper sees this when watching you walk, this is another indication that a strained glute med could have led to a strained gracilis.

If the cause of the groin region pain is found to be a strained gracilis, the muscles that need to be strengthened are the gluteus medius, the gluteus maximus, and the quads, and the gracilis needs to be stretched. The exercises to be performed are:

1. Gracilis Stretch (page 247)
2. Hip Abduction in sidelying or with a cable system (page 241)

3. Hip Extension with a resistance band or cable system (page 242)

4. Knee Extension (page 242)

Once the pain is resolved and the gracilis is back to its optimal length, do the following:

1. Hip Abduction in sidelying or with a cable system (page 241)

2. Straight Leg Deadlifts (page 246)

3. Hamstring Curl (page 240)

Possibility 2: Strained Sartorius

Another cause of groin pain is a strained sartorius muscle. The most obvious indicator that a strained sartorius muscle is the cause of the pain is if the pain starts near the outer hip and then comes into the groin region down the inner thigh and stops near the inner knee. This pattern follows the path of the sartorius muscle exactly.

Similar to the strained gracilis, the strained sartorius is often due to a strained glute med. Since the gluteus medius keeps the pelvis level, if it strains, it can cause the pelvis to drop on the opposite side of the body. This will cause muscles at the inner thigh on the side of the glute med strain to shorten and strain.

To determine if the pain in your groin is from a strained sartorius, we will do palpation, muscle testing, and posture analysis.

Palpation: The first test to identify a strained sartorius is palpation. Remember, our goal here is to find the muscle that is strained by eliciting pain through pressure. Press along the length of the sartorius muscle, starting at the ASIS (anterior superior iliac spine) on the front of the pelvis and moving down the thigh. The sartorius muscle sits just to the side of the inner border of the quads. A strained sartorius muscle will feel thick, almost ropelike. The final place to confirm that the sartorius has strained is at the attachment of the muscle to the lower leg bone, the tibia. The pes anserinus is a small bump just to the inside and bottom of the knee joint. This is where the sartorius attaches. If the sartorius is strained and you press on this point, it will hurt. If pain or knotting is felt anywhere along the muscle or at its attachment points, this is the first indicator that the groin pain is the result of a strained sartorius muscle.

Muscle Testing: The muscle test and the posture analysis described below are used to confirm the existence of a strained glute med, which could lead to a strained sartorius. To perform the muscle test, you'll need the help of someone else.

MUSCLE TESTING—GLUTEUS MEDIUS

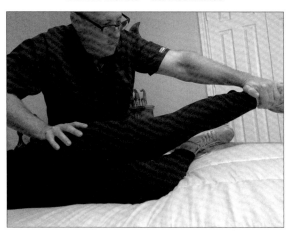

To test the strength of the glute med, lie down on a firm surface on your side. Raise your top leg a few inches, so it runs parallel to the floor. Make sure to keep it in line with your torso, not drifting forward or backward. Have your helper place one hand on your pelvis just above the hip joint and the other on your ankle. Try to push up at the ankle while the person tries to stop you. Then turn over and try the same test with the other leg. If the leg with the groin pain is found to be weaker, this is another indication that the cause of your groin pain is a sartorius strain caused by a strained glute med.

Posture Analysis: To do the posture analysis, stand in front of a mirror that can provide a full view of you from the front. Place your hands on the rim of your pelvis (most people consider this their hips) and see if one hand is higher than the other. If the glute med has strained, the pelvis on the opposite side will drop. Eventually, this will cause the lower back muscles to shorten in order to compensate, and those muscles will pull that same side up, causing it to be elevated. If the hip opposite your painful groin is elevated, this is another indicator that the sartorius may be strained because of a glute med strain.

STANDING POSTURE—NORMAL

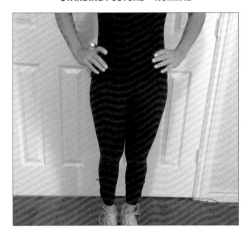

STANDING POSTURE—HIP HIKED

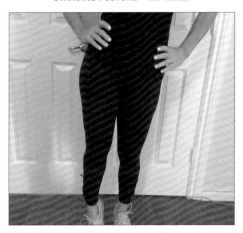

Finally, you can look at posture while walking. You will need someone to help you with this. Have the person stand behind you as you walk slowly away from him or her. As you are walking, the person should look to see if either of your hips dips down when taking a step through. He or she should watch the hip of the leg that is swinging forward just as the leg is lifted. Since the glute med plays an important role in stabilizing the pelvis, if it is weakened, the hip will dip as you walk.

WALKING POSTURE—NORMAL

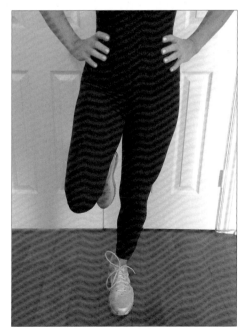

WALKING POSTURE—HIP DROP

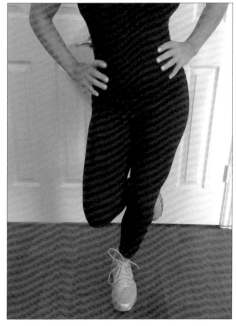

If the hips stay even when the affected leg is in motion (when the unaffected leg is stood on), but the hip dips when the unaffected leg is in motion (when the painful leg is stood on), this is an indication of a strained glute med, which could have led to a sartorius strain.

WALKING POSTURE—NORMAL   **WALKING POSTURE—SIDEBENT**

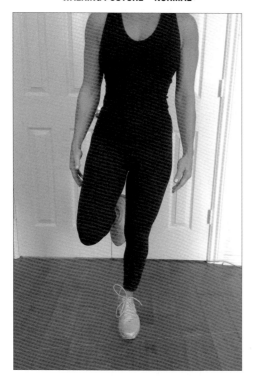 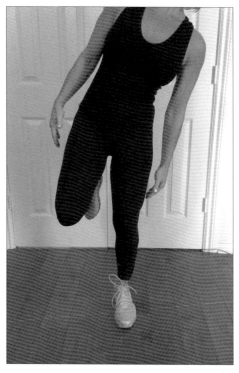

Another possible compensation that occurs when you have a strained glute med is that you bend to the side of the affected leg whenever that leg is stood on. By bending to the side of the injured leg, your body weight moves over the leg, which prevents the need for support of the weight by the strained glute med. If your helper sees this when watching you walk, this is another indication that a strained glute med could have led to a strained sartorius.

If the cause of the groin region pain is the result of a strained sartorius muscle, the muscles that need to be strengthened are the gluteus medius, gluteus maximus, and the quads. The sartorius will need to be lengthened. The exercises to be performed are:

1. Hip Abduction in sidelying or with a cable machine (page 241)
2. Hip Extension with a resistance bands or on a cable machine (page 242)
3. Knee Extension (page 242)
4. Sartorius Exercise (page 244)

Once the pain is resolved, do the following:

1. Hip Abduction in sidelying or with a cable machine (page 241)
2. Straight Leg Deadlifts (page 246)
3. Hamstring Curl (page 248)

CONCLUSION

The last 20 years have been an odyssey of discovery for me. Almost immediately in medical school I could tell that something didn't make sense in what I was being taught in terms of how pain is created and how I was supposed to resolve it. There was so much clinical evidence that the findings coming from MRIs and X-rays just didn't match the symptoms my patients were experiencing that I began to put together my own theories about treating pain, and thus created the Yass Method, which you've just learned about. I have had so much success treating pain by focusing on the muscular causes that I am ever frustrated by the medical establishment's treatment protocol.

After proving and re-proving this method with thousands of patients, I have utter confidence that this method is the cure for most chronic pain. I hope this book has given you an understanding of what pain is and the proper way to treat it—and not just the symptoms of pain, but the causes.

If you've been suffering from chronic pain, you know how it can destroy your life. You can't work, you can't parent, you can't have a normal life. But there's absolutely no reason you need to suffer physically, emotionally, and financially because of our faulty medical system. There is hope. There is freedom from pain. You just have to know where to look and when to question what the establishment tells you. The simplest way to do this is to understand if your symptoms match your diagnosis. My method looks at exactly this in order to identify which tissue is actually emitting pain. Once you know this, you can resolve your pain quickly and effectively by addressing the root cause—not just the symptoms.

For me, teaching this method is not simply about resolving pain; it is a moral directive to give people the chance to live their lives again. For years I have been asked why I am the only person who knows this system, and for years I have answered that I don't know. What I do know is that I was given the gift of learning it, and there has been no greater pleasure in my life than to pass this gift along to you. I am humbled to have had this opportunity. I have always believed and continue to believe that I am a simple servant to those I can help. Thank you. And may you live a long, healthy, pain-free life—just like you deserve to.

APPENDIX:
EXERCISES

This appendix will teach you how to perform the exercises to resolve pain associated with muscular causes. Before I describe the exercises, I would like to provide a basic understanding about strength training because so many people have misperceptions about what I'm talking about.

First of all, I don't want you to be afraid or concerned when I use the phrase *strength training.* The phrase simply implies that the technique we are going to use incorporates some form of resistance to make your muscles stronger. When you make the muscles stronger, you make sure they have the power to do the functional activities you are trying to perform. This will also prevent them from straining again, which is what brings about pain.

I am sure many of you have heard that simply moving your limbs with no resistance is an acceptable way to develop strength. But this is only true if you are doing these types of calisthenic movements instead of nothing. One of the core principles of developing strength is that the muscle gets stronger when it is forced to work against a resistance. Progressive resistance helps build more muscle, which makes the muscle stronger and more capable of performing functional activities. Your best chance of getting stronger with the intent to resolve and prevent pain, as well as enhance your functional capacity, will result from performing the proper exercises using some form of resistance.

Please do not think of strength training as bodybuilding. The goal of bodybuilding is to create aesthetic changes in the body. For the purpose of resolving pain, you will use much less resistance than bodybuilders use. In fact, you do not even need to use the same tools. Dumbbells or barbells are not necessary for this program, though I will describe their use along with weight-lifting equipment and resistance bands as options for creating the resistance that will be used in performing the exercises. The resistance bands vary in thickness and create varying levels of resistance (these can be purchased at most sporting-goods stores or online). For starting a program, try to find the least resistive bands so you can create a baseline of resistance you know you can use to complete the exercises. Then you can progress to more resistive bands.

For the past couple of years I have been performing home care, going to patients' homes to treat them. Because of the nature of the job, which requires me to travel from house to house, I needed a simple lightweight method of creating resistance for the patients I treat. The use of elastic resistance bands has been highly successful in this role. The bands come in different resistances, which allows me to progressively build strength in the patients until they are pain-free and fully functional. Luckily for me—and for you—these bands are widely available, and they're not that expensive. Don't be concerned about the type of device you use to create the resistance to perform the required exercises. Just recognize that the right resistance used with the right exercise performed correctly is the path to resolving your pain. The choice of which method of resistance to use is yours.

The other choice you'll need to make is if you want to do these exercises at home or at a gym. The two considerations to look at for this choice are (a) if you feel comfortable at a gym and (b) whether you want to buy your own equipment or simply use the gym's.

No matter where you do the exercise, the key to success is threefold:

1. Know which muscles need to be strengthened. This is the work you did in Part II of the book.

2. Understand how to perform the techniques correctly, which I teach you in this appendix.

3. Incorporate the correct resistance to make the affected muscle(s) stronger, which we will also discuss here.

You might think that strength training is complicated or you may know people who got hurt while trying to strengthen their muscles. To ease this fear, I can only speak to my understanding and my experience in treating patients up to the age of 102. Strength training techniques should be simple and safe to perform. If the technique seems complex to perform, it is most likely dangerous and should not be used. None of the exercises included in this book fall into that category.

The strength training techniques that start on page 234 work to isolate muscles to make them stronger. This means that the rest of your body, which is not being used to perform the exercise, should be fully stable. This makes loss of balance, a common concern, out of the question.

Another question I often get asked is: "If I have pain doing normal activities, how is it possible for me to do strength training without pain?" With the exercises in these pages, this shouldn't be a worry either. The pain you often feel is associated with functional activities like walking or climbing stairs. These activities require a variety of muscles to work at the same time. Once a muscle strains and emits pain, performing the activities continues to create pain. With the strength training we will be doing, we are isolating muscles. We are not performing tasks that require multiple muscles to work and therefore lead to strained muscles that emit pain.

The final, and perhaps biggest, concern people have when thinking about starting a strength training program is that they don't know what to do or how to begin. The great part of this book is that all these questions are answered. You've already identified the muscles that need to be worked, and in the descriptions of the exercises, which start on page 234, I explain the rest. This is a strength training road map. You should not need to learn any information that is not provided in this book.

In this section, every exercise required by this book is presented—both in text and in images. I am a big proponent of pictures because I believe in the idea that a picture is worth a thousand words. The start and finish pictures in the following pages show you the boundaries of each exercise. If you simply move from the start position presented to the finish position presented, you should be performing the exercises safely and effectively. Add the written cues to point out key aspects of each exercise and you should be more than prepared to perform the exercises correctly.

How do you know what the proper resistance is to cause a muscle to strengthen without straining it? To figure this out, I use the scale of perceived exertion with my patients.

The perceived exertion scale works like this: You perform a set of exercise for strengthening a muscle and try to pick a number from 1 to 10 determining how much effort you felt you needed to finish the set. A 10 describes the feeling of tearing a muscle, while a 1 describes the feeling of doing nothing. If you are just starting strength training for the first time, I suggest that you work at a level of 5. This implies that you are working at 50 percent of your maximum effort. This is a very safe level, meaning that there is almost no chance of straining a muscle.

You can stay with this level of effort for a few sessions. Once you feel you have become comfortable performing the exercises, you can bump up your effort load to 80 percent. This is considered the most effective effort level to strengthen muscles while avoiding straining. In fact, this is the level recommended by the American Heart Association, the Centers for Disease Control and Prevention, and the American College of Sports Medicine in its *Guidelines for Exercise Testing and Prescription*. The only group with a different effort level recommended is children from eight years old to puberty. They should work out at an effort level of 5, or 50 percent of their maximum effort (moderate effort).

Now that you know how to identify the right resistance, the next question is how many repetitions should be performed and how many sets. The general theory of strength training exercise is to perform three sets of ten repetitions.

In performing ten repetitions, the resistance should be enough to cause a muscle to grow without the chance of straining or leading to bad technique in performing the exercise. More advanced individuals who have been strength training for a while might use a repetition count less than ten. Since you are performing fewer repetitions in a set, this would allow you to lift more weight over the course of the set. This would speed up the process of causing muscles to get stronger by adapting to more resistance at a faster rate. But I think that ten repetitions per set is a good standard for most people who are trying to get stronger. For those who have heard that you should be performing 15 repetitions or more in an attempt to get stronger, let me explain why this theory won't work.

When a muscle contracts it starts to develop lactic acid, which inhibits the ability of the muscle to contract. The more lactic acid develops, the less muscle mass is available to perform the exercise. So the more repetitions in a set, the more chance there is for lactic acid to build up. For those who are performing these high repetition counts, what you will notice is that as you reach these later repetitions, you experience burning in the muscle. You will also find that it gets harder and harder to complete the repetition. The reason for this is that you have less and less muscle mass available because of the lactic acid buildup that is occurring. The only way to make a muscle get stronger is to make it adapt to greater and greater resistance. This can only occur when you have the maximal amount of muscle mass available, which means that the repetition counts must be kept fairly low so not too much lactic acid builds up and impedes the muscle's ability. This is why I never have a patient perform more than ten repetitions in a set.

As for the number of sets, the standard has pretty much always been three. If there is a time constraint that inhibits you from performing three sets of each exercise and you can only get in two sets of each exercise, that is okay.

The next thing we need to cover is how much time you should take between each set. Why is this important? Again, it's due to lactic acid. Just as performing higher repetition counts can cause a buildup of lactic acid, so can not waiting long enough in between the sets of exercises. Lactic acid continues to build up in a muscle until the muscle relaxes. At that point, the blood vessels, which constrict during exercise, open and remove the lactic acid. To allow enough time for this to happen, you should rest about 45 seconds between sets if you are working at 50 percent of your maximum effort. If you are working out at 80 percent of your maximum effort, wait for 60 to 90 seconds between sets. A simple gauge to know if you are waiting long enough is that performing each successive set should take the same amount of effort. If the second set is harder than the first, or if you can't perform as many repetitions, you didn't wait long enough.

All right. You're almost ready to get started. There's just one thing left. How often should you perform the routine? The answer is no more than two or three times a week. Why? Because when you are strength training, you are actually causing small breakdowns in the muscle that need to heal in order to strengthen the muscle. For 24 to 48 hours after you work out, your muscles are rebuilding and growing. If you work out during this healing period, the muscle is susceptible to strain. No muscle should be strengthened more than three times a week.

The stretching exercises, which start on page 247, however, should be performed every day. Each stretch is held for about 20 seconds and is performed in sets of two. The stretches are an adjunct to the strengthening exercises and can help increase the speed at which your pain is resolved. Stretching is not a replacement for strengthening and certainly has a lesser ability to resolve muscle weakness or imbalance.

So there you have it. I have given you the exercises to perform and how to perform them. I have shown you how to pick the right resistance. I have told you how many repetitions to perform and how many sets of each exercise to perform. I have told you how long to rest in between the sets of your exercise and how often to work out. You should have everything you need to begin to resolve your pain.

STRENGTHENING EXERCISES

Upper Body (arranged alphabetically by exercise)

External Rotation (rotator cuff): You can do this exercise using a dumbbell or resistance band. With the elbow supported at the end of a surface so that the elbow is just below shoulder height, the elbow should be maintained at a 90-degree angle through the whole motion. The elbow of the arm performing the exercise should be in a line with both shoulders (if the elbow is in front of this line, the rotator cuff will have difficulty performing the exercise). The start position is with the forearm facing about 20 degrees below parallel. The resistance is pulled upward until the forearm is facing about 20 degrees above parallel. Then return to the start position. This is an exercise where people seem to go through too much range of motion. If excessive range of motion is performed, there is a chance of straining the rotator cuff.

START	FINISH	START	FINISH

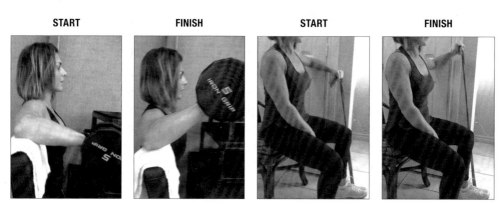

Internal Rotation (strengthens the pecs, lats, and teres major and lengthens the rotator cuff): You can do this exercise using a cable system or resistance band. With the elbow supported at the end of a surface so that the elbow is just below shoulder height, the elbow should be maintained at a 90-degree angle through the whole motion. The elbow of the arm performing the exercise should be in line with both shoulders (if the elbow is in front of this line, the rotator cuff will have difficulty performing the exercise). The start position is with the forearm facing about 20 degrees above parallel. The resistance is pulled downward until the forearm is facing about 20 degrees below parallel. Then return to the start position. This is an exercise where people seem to go through too much range of motion. If excessive range of motion is performed, there is a chance of straining the rotator cuff.

START	FINISH	START	FINISH

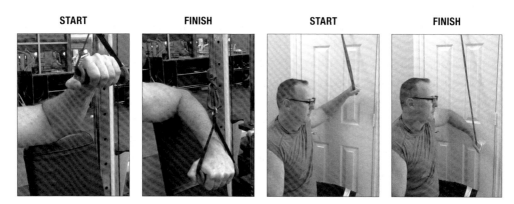

Lat Pulldown with Neutral Bar or Elastic Band (interscapular muscles: mid-traps and rhomboids): Leaning back with an angle at the hip of about 30 degrees, reach up for the bar or elastic band so that the start position begins with the arms nearly straight and the elbows just unlocked. Pull the mechanism down keeping your arms wide and bringing the elbows just below shoulder height and slightly behind the line of the shoulders. At this point, you should feel the shoulder blades squeeze together (the elbows will barely reach behind the line of the shoulders if performing this exercise correctly); then return to the start position. If the elbows start to drop so they are lower than the shoulders, you are using the incorrect muscles to perform the exercise.

START	FINISH	START	FINISH

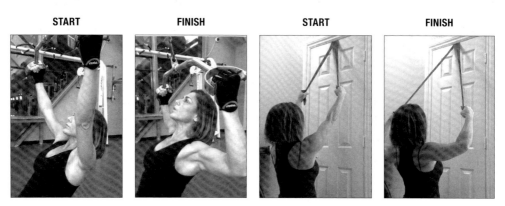

Lower Trap Exercise (lower trapezius muscle): This has become one of the exercises I feel is critical to achieving complete functional capacity of the shoulder. To perform this exercise, sit in a sturdy chair and lean back slightly—about 10 degrees. This will prevent the resistance from pulling you forward. Start with your arm halfway between pointing straight forward and pointing straight to the side, with your hand at shoulder height and your elbow just unlocked. Begin to raise the resistance until the arm reaches about 130 to 140 degrees (about the height of the ear). Then return to the start position at shoulder height. Make sure you are sitting and are supported with a chair back if possible. You want to be leaning back about 10 degrees to prevent the resistance from pulling you forward.

START	FINISH	START	FINISH

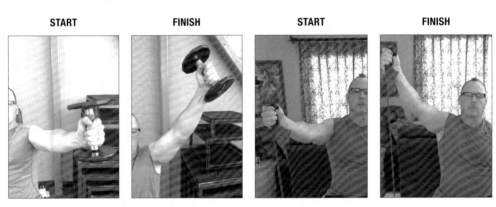

Posterior Deltoids (posterior deltoids): Stand with your feet more than shoulder width apart, knees slightly bent and your butt pushed behind you. Your weight should be mostly on your heels. Hold the resistance in front of your thighs with your palms facing in and your elbows unlocked. Begin to move the resistance out to your side from the shoulders like a pendulum. Go out until you feel the shoulder blades start to move inward (about 60 degrees), and then return to the beginning position.

START	FINISH	FINISH (FRONT VIEW)

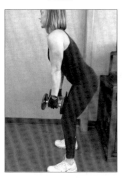 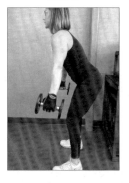 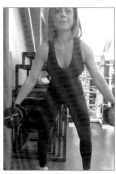

START	FINISH

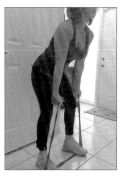 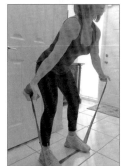

Protraction Punch (serratus anterior): Lying on your back with your feet supported on the floor, raise the arm performing the exercise so the hand and resistance are directly over the shoulder, with the elbow just unlocked. Then raise the arm slightly using a slow punching movement. This will raise your shoulder slightly off the surface you are lying on. Make sure you do not rotate your torso to try to get more range of motion. Your back doesn't move at all during this exercise; just the shoulder is being raised off the surface. Once the appropriate height is reached, slowly return to the start position.

START	FINISH	FINISH (CLOSEUP)

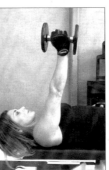 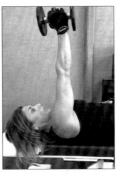 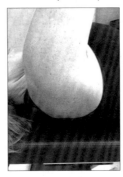

START	FINISH

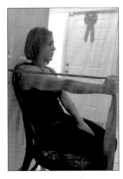 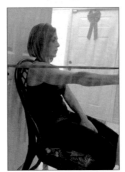

Skull Crushers (triceps, single and both arms): There are a multitude of exercises to perform to strengthen the triceps. The reason this is the most effective is because it puts the long head of the triceps in the optimal position. The long head of the triceps is the only part of the triceps muscle that passes the shoulder joint. Therefore, it is the only part of the muscle that can affect the position of the arm bone in the shoulder joint. The exercise can be performed with one arm or both, depending on whether your pain is associated with one side or requires both arms to be strengthened to resolve it. To perform the exercise, lie on your back with your feet supported on the floor. Start with the arms straight up in front of you, in line with your shoulders and the elbows just unlocked. Keeping the upper arm in place, begin to bend the elbows lowering the forearms so the hands and resistance are moving toward your forehead. Once the elbow reaches 90 degrees, return to the start position. Make sure not to lock the elbows at the top of the motion.

START	FINISH	START (BILATERAL)	FINISH (BILATERAL)

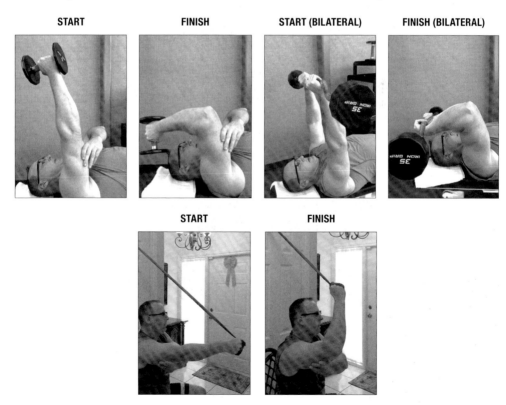

START	FINISH

Lower Body (arranged alphabetically by exercise)

Dorsiflexion (anterior tibialis): With the leg supported on a surface and the ankle and foot hanging off, attach the resistance so that it is supported on the front of the foot in the mid-foot region. Start with the ankle angled about 30 degrees forward, then pull the ankle toward the face about 10 degrees beyond perpendicular. Then return to the start position.

START	FINISH	START	FINISH

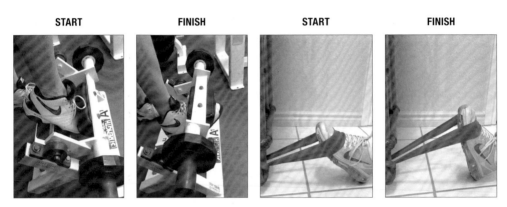

Hamstring Curl (hamstrings): In a seated position place the resistance at the back of the ankle. Make sure you are supported in the seat. Begin with the exercising leg pointing straight out with the knee unlocked. Begin to bend the knee until it reaches 90 degrees. Then return to the start position. To isolate the hamstrings better, have the toes of the exercising leg pointing toward the face as the exercise is being performed. In the case of using a seated Hamstring Curl machine, make sure the pivot point of the machine is aligned with the knee joint.

START	FINISH	START	FINISH

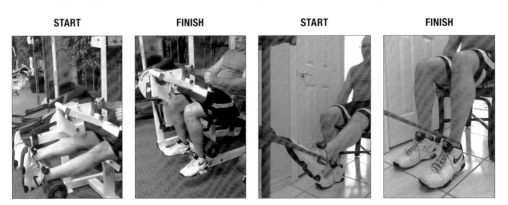

Hip Abduction (gluteus medius): This exercise can be performed either lying on your side or standing. To do this exercise correctly, make sure you do not go too far when moving your leg outward. There is a false sense that more range of motion is better, but in this case too much range of motion means you are using the lower back muscle to create the motion, not the gluteus medius (hip muscle). The gluteus medius muscle can only move the leg out to the point where it is parallel with the hip joint. Any outward motion beyond that is created by the lower back muscle.

To do the exercise, lie on your side with the knee of the bottom leg bent and the top leg straight. The top leg should run in a continuous line from the torso. If the leg is angled in front of the torso, you are using a different muscle than the gluteus medius. Start to raise the top leg off the supporting leg until your leg is parallel with the floor. Try to turn the leg in slightly so the heel is the first part of the foot that is moving. This puts the gluteus medius in the optimal position to raise the leg. Once your leg reaches parallel to the floor, begin to lower back onto the supporting leg.

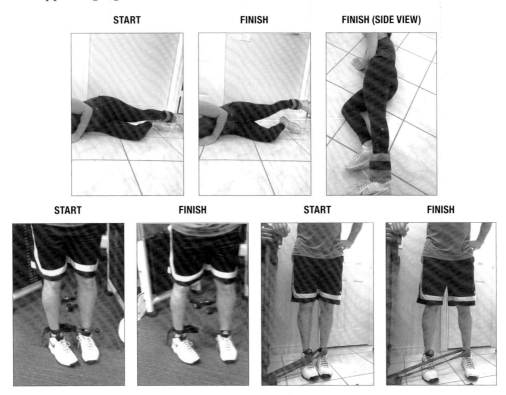

241

This exercise can be performed utilizing the same technique but standing with a resistance band or cable column in a gym setting. In this instance, you will simply pull the leg to the side until your ankle is in line with the hip slightly against the resistance.

Hip Extension (gluteus maximus): In a sitting or standing position, place the resistance behind your knee. Start with the hip flexed to about 60 degrees. If you are sitting, bring the knee down to the surface you are sitting on. If you are standing, bring the knee about 10 degrees behind the hip. Then return to the start position. If standing, make sure your back is rounded and the knee of the leg you are standing on is unlocked.

START	FINISH	START	FINISH

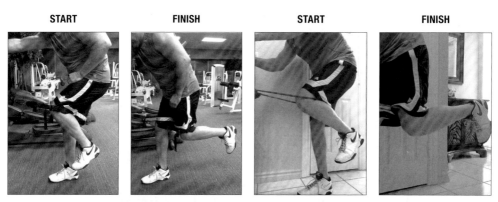

Knee Extension (quads): In a seated position, place the resistance around the front of the ankle. Make sure the foot of the opposite leg is on the floor and you are supported in a seat. Begin with the knee bent to 90 degrees, then straighten the knee until it is almost locked. Then return the leg to the start position. Make sure the thigh of the leg that is being exercised remains on the seat and does not rise with the lower leg as the exercise is performed.

START	FINISH	START	FINISH

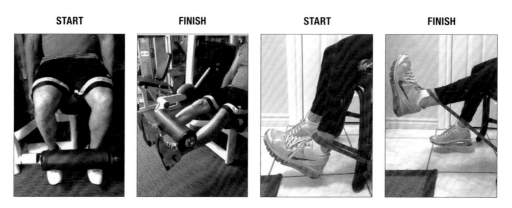

Leg Press: I am actually not a big fan of the Leg Press. When performing this exercise, there is a tendency for the lower back to become rounded as the knees are brought toward the chest. This creates a situation where the spine is no longer supporting the lower back; only the lower back muscles are, which makes them more likely to strain. Only perform the Leg Press if you have a balance issue preventing you from doing Squats or Lunges.

To do the Leg Press, place the feet on the plate fairly high so that you are creating a 90-degree angle at the knees and a 90-degree angle at the hips. The plate should not move any farther toward you during the motion of the exercise. Then start to push the plate away from you using your feet with the majority of the force going through the heels. Too much force through the balls of the feet and you will be utilizing a lot of your calves to move the resistance. Move the plate away from you until the knees reach an unlocked position. Then return to the start position. If at all possible, try to keep a slight arch in the lower back during the exercise.

START **FINISH**

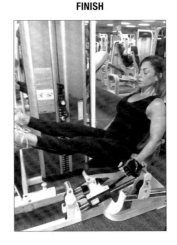

Lunges: Lunges require a bit of balance to complete, so please don't do these if you feel unsteady in any way. You might want to perform this exercise without using extra weight (so you can grab on to something during the motion); however, using resistance in each hand will improve your balance because the weight on either side of your body actually helps stabilize you.

To do this exercise, spread your feet a little wider than shoulder width apart. Then place one foot in front of you and one foot behind, keeping them the same width apart. The whole foot of the front leg will be on the floor, while only the ball of the foot behind will be on the floor. Next, lower the back knee toward the floor. The front knee will bend, but make sure it does not end up in front of the front foot. Lower yourself until the front thigh is parallel to the floor. Then return to the start position.

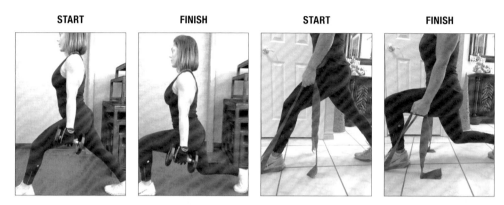

START   **FINISH**   **START**   **FINISH**

Sartorius Exercise (lengthens the sartorius muscle): Make sure you are holding on to a sturdy object when performing this exercise to help you with your balance. In a standing position, place the resistance around the back of the ankle of the leg to be strengthened. Start by rotating the hip of the leg performing the exercise so the toes are pointing inward slightly. Then begin to place the foot of the exercising leg behind the foot of the leg you are standing on. Once the foot of the exercising leg is placed down on the floor behind the other leg, return it to the start position. Make sure the resistance is appropriate so you can get your exercising foot behind the foot that you are standing on. You want to use a resistance that helps lengthen the sartorius, but, because there is a balance element to this exercise, caution should be used in determining the right resistance.

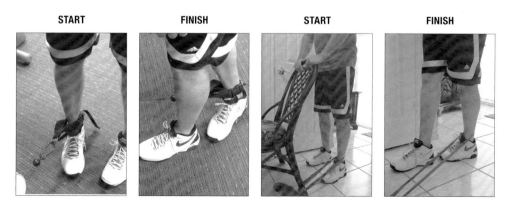

START   **FINISH**   **START**   **FINISH**

Squats (quads primarily): The main muscle that performs the squat is the quads (front thigh muscle), not the hamstrings or butt muscles. To perform the squat, start with your feet a little more than shoulder width apart and your toes pointed outward. The knees are unlocked and the butt is pushed backward slightly. The resistance is held in the hands, with the hands at the side of the body. The key to performing a squat properly is to envision that you are sitting down in a chair. The butt moves backward as the shoulders move forward. The knees should remain as close to over the ankles as possible. Remember that a deep knee bend is when you go down and the knee moves forward but the hips stay over the ankles. In a squat the knees stay over the ankles and the butt goes backward as the shoulders move forward. The goal is to sit down far enough, until your thighs are parallel to the ground, and then return to the start position.

| START | FINISH | START | FINISH |

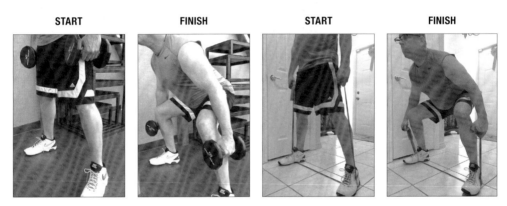

For some, balance might be an issue. If so, don't go so far down. As you gain confidence and strength, you can work your way to the point where your thighs are parallel to the ground. You can also put a chair behind you. This will not only help you visualize the idea of sitting down in a chair; it will also catch you if you lose your balance.

Standing Calf Raises: To perform this exercise, start with your feet shoulder width apart, holding the weights at your side. Bring your heels off the floor, rising up on the balls of your feet. Then return to the start position. Keep the knees unlocked during the movement. This exercise can also be performed with a resistance band by placing the band under the balls of your feet and pulling the bands tight with your hands, thus creating resistance, before raising your heels.

START	FINISH	START	FINISH

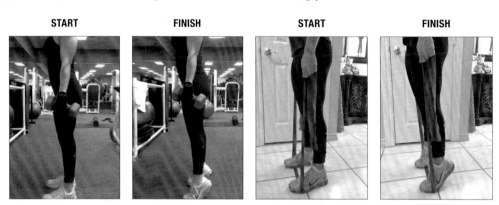

Straight Leg Deadlifts (gluteus maximus and hamstrings): Start with your feet a little more than shoulder width apart and your toes pointing slightly out. You should be standing straight with your knees unlocked and your butt pushed back slightly. Hold the resistance in front of your thighs. Bend from the hips, keeping your back straight while looking out in front of you, and begin to lower the resistance down your legs. Make sure your knees don't bend and the motion is coming from your hips. As you move down, you should feel the weight shift to your heels. When you begin to feel tightness at the back of your thighs, begin to straighten back up to the start position. There is no specific point to come down to on the leg. To determine how far down to go, reach a tightness at the back of your thighs. Make sure your back remains straight, not rounded. If it's rounded, you can strain your back and you will also go down farther than you could with a straight back.

START   **FINISH**   **START**   **FINISH**

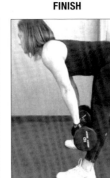 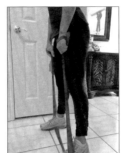 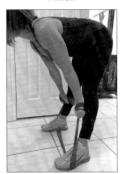

STRETCHING EXERCISES (ARRANGED ALPHABETICALLY)

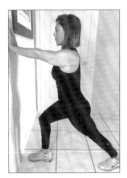

Calf Stretch: Stand in front of a wall. With your arms straight, place your hands on the wall. Keeping your feet hip width apart, bend one knee and step the other foot slightly back. The calf of the back leg will be stretched. Make sure the whole foot stays on the floor during the stretch. Keeping the knee of the front leg bent, move your torso forward so more of your body weight is on the front leg. Continue moving forward until you feel a stretch in the back calf. Once you feel the stretch, hold it for 20 seconds and then return to the start position.

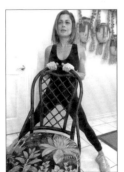

Gracilis Stretch: Stand next to a wall or an object that you can use to support yourself. Start to move your legs out to the side, spreading slowly until you start to feel a stretch at the inner thighs. Make sure the knees are unlocked when performing this action. Hold the stretch for 20 seconds and then return to the start position. As for many people, you will not get very far before you feel a stretch. That is okay. Just continue with the process and over time you will be able to stretch farther. The key is to perform this stretch slowly, only spreading your legs enough to feel a mild stretch.

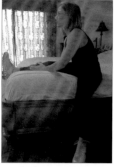

Hamstring Stretch: Sitting on a surface with the leg to be stretched pointing in front of you and the other leg hanging off the side, place your hands on the thigh of the leg to be stretched. Make sure your back stays in a straight position and you don't hunch. Start to move your chest toward the leg out in front of you, keeping the knee unlocked and the toes pointing forward, away from your face. Continue to move the chest toward the leg until you feel a stretch at the back of the thigh. Once you feel the stretch, hold it for 20 seconds and then return to the start position. You may not go too far before feeling the tightness at the back of the thigh. That's okay; you will improve over time.

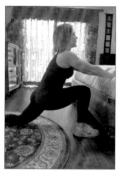

Hip Flexor Stretch: Kneel down on one knee next to an object like a chair or couch that will help you balance when performing this exercise. The leg you are kneeling on is the one with the hip flexor that will be stretched. Slowly move the opposite leg in front of you with the foot on the floor and the knee bent. Begin to move the pelvis forward with your torso upright so you start to move closer to the front foot. You will begin to get a stretch at the upper thigh region of the leg you are kneeling on. Once a comfortable stretch is felt, hold it for 20 seconds.

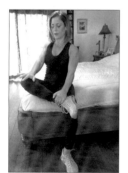

ITB Stretch: Start by sitting in a chair with both feet on the floor. Place the ankle of the leg you are trying to stretch on the opposite knee. Put both hands on the knee of the leg you are trying to stretch and slowly press the knee down toward the floor, feeling a stretch at the outer thigh anywhere from the hip to the knee. Once a light stretch is felt, hold the position for 20 seconds. Then return to the start position.

Some people's ITB may be too tight to be able to put the ankle on the opposite knee. If this is the case, start by placing the ankle halfway up the shin and holding it there with one hand while pressing down on the knee. This can be progressed until the ankle can finally be placed on the opposite knee to perform the stretch.

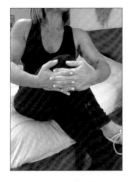

Piriformis Stretch: Sitting in a chair or on a bed, place the ankle of the leg to be stretched on the bent knee of the opposite leg. If the ankle cannot be placed on the knee, place it as high up on the shin as possible. Then grab the knee of the leg to be stretched with both hands. Pull the knee toward the opposite shoulder until a stretch is felt in the butt. Once you feel the stretch, hold it for 20 seconds and then return to the start position. This stretch can be used to diminish sciatic symptoms for short-term relief.

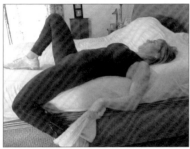

Quad Stretch: Lie on a surface with the leg to be stretched hanging off the side and the other leg on the surface with the knee bent and the foot on the surface. Next, place a towel around the ankle of the leg to be stretched in order to give you something to hold on to. Grab the towel and slowly begin to bend the knee toward the butt until a stretch is felt in the front of the thigh. Once you feel the stretch, hold it for 20 seconds and then return to the start position. Make sure your back does not arch when performing the stretch. This is a very stable position for stretching the quad, and most people should be able to do this versus standing up and pulling the heel toward the butt, which is a commonly suggested quad stretch.

NOTES

1. Ginevra L. Liptan, "Fascia: A missing link in our understanding of the pathology of fibromyalgia," *Journal of Bodywork & Movement Therapies* 14, no. 1 (January 2010): 3–12.

2. Gina Kolata, "Sports Medicine Said to Overuse M.R.I.'s," *The New York Times,* October 28, 2011.

3. J. Bruce Moseley et al., "A Controlled Trial of Arthroscopic Surgery for Osteoarthritis of the Knee," *New England Journal of Medicine* 347 (July 11, 2002): 81–88.

4. "When Is Back Surgery a Good Idea?", *Arthritis Advisor,* July 2011, http://www.arthritis-advisor.com/issues/10_7/features/733-1.html.

5. Maureen C. Jensen et al., "Magnetic resonance imaging of the lumbar spine in people without back pain," *New England Journal of Medicine* 331, no. 2 (July 14, 1994): 69-73.

ACKNOWLEDGMENTS

First I would like to thank Lauren Levine. Lauren came to me due to pain she was experiencing that was unresolved by a surgery. Her father had seen me in some local media and suggested she see me to resolve her pain. Within just a couple of weeks her pain was essentially gone. After having her pain resolved so quickly and easily and after hearing stories from other patients she met while being treated at my facility at the time, she felt compelled to help me reach a broader audience and to do so she would lead me to PBS.

Next I would like to thank Bob Marty. Bob is a tireless worker. He has been producing shows for PBS for over 25 years. With Laruen's introduction, Bob and I began our relationship. I think Bob sensed something very unusual and passionate about me and this method I had created. He seemed in step with me regarding its reach and importance. It wasn't easy to get the PBS special produced and on air, but Bob never gave up and he showed me that he was as committed to me as I was to getting people around the world the information that will end their plague of living with chronic pain. He has helped lead me to international exposure and for that I am deeply grateful.

I must thank Reid Tracy. Clearly, he is a man with vision. Bob approached Reid about working together for the first time regarding my PBS special and this book. Bob gave Reid my first book and a copy of my PBS test show. He seemed to almost instantly get it. I was addressing the biggest health issue affecting people worldwide and he knew that his company had the infrastructure that could help reach those people. I am honored to be working with such esteemed gentlemen as Bob Marty and Reid Tracy.

To Laura Gray, thank you for taking four hundred pages of text and turning it into a cohesive, thoughtful, and useful book. At times I get so caught up in trying to present the facts, I lose track of what people can understand and interpret. You assisted me in creating a book that will help resolve the pain of millions.

None of my success would have been possible without my wife, Lisa. She has seen me through the darkest days of this journey and helped me want to continue when things looked so bleak. I am eternally in her debt. She is as much to thank for getting my method to people around the world as I am. And to my daughter, Natalya, she is our light. She makes waking up every day a joy. There is an energy that flows from her that is pure goodness. I have used that energy to help me overcome the negative emotions that existed when things were not going so well for me. To my wife and my daughter, my success is a tribute to the both of you.

ABOUT THE AUTHOR

Dr. Mitchell Yass has spent the past 20 years developing his method of diagnosing and treating the cause, not the symptom, of pain and believes that this is the future of pain relief. He is currently treating patients in Florida utilizing his unique method, is the author of *Overpower Pain: The Strength Training Program That Stops Pain Without Drugs or Surgery,* and was host of the radio show *Stop the Pain! I Want My Life Back.* He has written articles for various publications, including *Advance for Physical Therapists and PT Assistants, Bottom Line Health,* and *Cure-Back-Pain.org,* and he has been featured on numerous radio shows. Learn more at www.mitchellyass.com.

HAY HOUSE TITLES OF RELATED INTEREST

YOU CAN HEAL YOUR LIFE, the movie, starring Louise Hay & Friends
(available as a 1-DVD program and an expanded 2-DVD set)
Watch the trailer at: www.LouiseHayMovie.com

THE SHIFT, the movie,
starring Dr. Wayne W. Dyer
(available as a 1-DVD program and an expanded 2-DVD set)
Watch the trailer at: www.DyerMovie.com

*GODDESSES NEVER AGE: The Secret Prescription for Radiance,
Vitality, and Well-Being,* by Christiane Northrup, M.D.

*TALK RX: Five Steps to Honest Conversations That Create
Connection, Health, and Happiness,* by Neha Sangwan, M.D.

All of the above are available at your local bookstore,
or may be ordered by contacting Hay House (see next page).

We hope you enjoyed this Hay House book. If you'd like
to receive our online catalog featuring additional information
on Hay House books and products, or if you'd like to find
out more about the Hay Foundation, please contact:

Hay House, Inc., P.O. Box 5100, Carlsbad, CA 92018-5100
(760) 431-7695 or (800) 654-5126
(760) 431-6948 (fax) or (800) 650-5115 (fax)
www.hayhouse.com® • www.hayfoundation.org

Published and distributed in Australia by: Hay House Australia Pty. Ltd., 18/36 Ralph St.,
Alexandria NSW 2015 • *Phone:* 612-9669-4299 • *Fax:* 612-9669-4144 • www.hayhouse.com.au

Published and distributed in the United Kingdom by: Hay House UK, Ltd., Astley House,
33 Notting Hill Gate, London W11 3JQ • *Phone:* 44-20-3675-2450 • *Fax:* 44-20-3675-2451
www.hayhouse.co.uk

Published and distributed in the Republic of South Africa by:
Hay House SA (Pty), Ltd., P.O. Box 990, Witkoppen 2068 • info@hayhouse.co.za

Published in India by: Hay House Publishers India, Muskaan Complex, Plot No. 3, B-2, Vasant
Kunj, New Delhi 110 070 • *Phone:* 91-11-4176-1620 • *Fax:* 91-11-4176-1630 • www.hayhouse.co.in

Distributed in Canada by: Raincoast Books, 2440 Viking Way, Richmond, B.C. V6V 1N2
Phone: 1-800-663-5714 • *Fax:* 1-800-565-3770 • www.raincoast.com

Take Your Soul on a Vacation

Visit www.HealYourLife.com® to regroup, recharge,
and reconnect with your own magnificence.
Featuring blogs, mind-body-spirit news, and life-changing
wisdom from Louise Hay and friends.

Visit www.HealYourLife.com today!

Free e-newsletters
from Hay House, the Ultimate
Resource for Inspiration

Be the first to know about Hay House's dollar deals, free downloads, special offers, affirmation cards, giveaways, contests, and more!

Get exclusive excerpts from our latest releases and videos from *Hay House Present Moments*.

Enjoy uplifting personal stories, how-to articles, and healing advice, along with videos and empowering quotes, within *Heal Your Life*.

Have an inspirational story to tell and a passion for writing? Sharpen your writing skills with insider tips from *Your Writing Life*.

Sign Up Now!

Get inspired, educate yourself, get a complimentary gift, and share the wisdom!

http://www.hayhouse.com/newsletters.php

Visit www.hayhouse.com to sign up today!

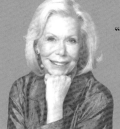
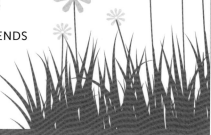